The
Advanced Mediterranean Diet

2nd Edition

Please visit us on the Internet
to find updated information, answers to
frequently asked questions, printable documents
(e.g., grocery shopping list. daily logs), and more:

http://AdvancedMediterraneanDiet.com

Join the discussion at Dr. Parker's
Advanced Mediterranean Diet Blog:

http://AdvancedMediterraneandDiet.com/blog/

Also by Steve Parker, M.D.:

*Conquer Diabetes and Prediabetes: The Low-Carb
Mediterranean Diet*

http://DiabeticMediterraneanDiet.com

Dr. Parker's current research interest is application
of the Paleolithic diet as therapy for diabetes. Follow
his progress at:

http://PaleoDiabetic.com

2nd Edition

The
Advanced Mediterranean Diet

Lose Weight   Feel Better   Live Longer

Steve Parker, M.D.

pxHealth

First edition published 2007
Newly revised and updated edition 2012
ISBN 978-0-9791284-6-2
Library of Congress Control Number: 2011915815

Published by pxHealth
PO Box 27276
Scottsdale, Arizona 85255 USA
Phone: (480) 695-3192
Web: http://pxHealth.com

Publisher's Cataloging-in-Publication data

Parker, Steven Paul.
    The advanced Mediterranean diet : lose weight, feel better, live longer, 2nd edition / Steve Parker, M.D.
        p. cm.
    ISBN   978-0-9791284-6-2
    Includes bibliographical references and index.

1. Diet --Mediterranean Region. 2. Cooking, Mediterranean. 3. Weight loss. 4. Diet therapy --Mediterranean Region. 5. Obesity --Prevention 6. Insulin resistance --Diet therapy. 7. Low-carbohydrate diet. 8. Dietary Carbohydrates --Administration & dosage --Popular Works. I. Title.

RM222.2 .P37 2012
613.2/5 –dc22   2011915815

CONTENTS

To those working
in the weight-management field
who value truth above personal profit

Disclaimer

Preface to the Newly Revised and Updated Second Edition

WHY A NEW EDITION?

Since publication of the first edition in 2007, medical and nutrition scientists have made several watershed advances in our understanding of optimal nutrition and weight management. This second edition incorporates that new knowledge, along with other important eye-opening research results.

The most astounding new scientific findings are that the saturated fat and total fat content of our diets do not cause or contribute to heart and vascular disease. The same is true for cholesterol in our food. In other words, foods that contain fat, saturated fat, and cholesterol don't cause us to have heart attacks, strokes, or hardening of the arteries (atherosclerosis), or high blood pressure. These statements apply to a large majority of people, although there may be rare exceptions.

This new knowledge, which is accepted by most experts in medical nutrition science, runs counter to popular thought and teaching of the last four decades. At the same time, it's true that the information hasn't yet trickled down to many physicians and dietitians working in the trenches of clinical care. The scientific supporting literature is listed at the back of the book in the Selected References section.

The second earth-shaking development is the discovery that certain carbohydrates are particularly prone to make us gain excess fat weight, and that avoiding those carbohydrates can be especially helpful in weight management. This is best demonstrated by numerous scientific studies that document more successful weight loss in dieters who drastically reduce consumption of carbohydrates, at least for the short term. The idea that carbohydrates are uniquely fattening applies to a majority of people, but certainly not all. The scientific supporting literature is listed at the back of the book in the Selected References section.

These advances led me to design a very-low-carbohydrate version of the Mediterranean diet, included herein as the Ketogenic Mediterranean Diet. The original *Advanced Mediterranean Diet* is also here, modified to allow more total and saturated fat. You choose which diet you wish to follow, depending on your needs, proclivities, and personal metabolism. Or use both diets at different times.

The first edition of the Advanced Mediterranean Diet noted numerous health benefits to eating Mediterranean style, including increased longevity and reduced rates of heart disease, stroke, dementia and cancer of the colon, breast, prostate, and uterus.

Studies published over the last five years have expanded the list of health benefits even further, to include prevention of type 2 diabetes and stomach cancer, for example.

To lose excess weight, you've got to exercise a lot, right? That's now old school thought, and not really true. The latest research tells us that, in general, exercise contributes only minimally to successful real-world weight loss. "Real world" as opposed to The Biggest Loser TV show. And what's a minimal contribution to weight loss? About 10%. What about exercise's role in long-term weight management? That's a whole 'nother can o' worms.

THE KEY TO WEIGHT MANAGEMENT

I will assume that you're overweight and reading this book to lose weight. My goal is to share with you the information that has helped my personal patients lose weight effectively, safely, and permanently. Reduction of excess body fat has been particularly critical for my patients with diabetes, high blood pressure, heart problems, strokes, low back pain, and lower limb arthritis. Even if you're essentially healthy, you may need to lose 10 to 50 pounds (4.5 to 23 kg) in order to feel and look your best.

The standard medical approach to weight loss too often is:

- a five-minute lecture on proper eating and exercise habits
- presentation of a confusing, unrealistic, calorie-restricted diet pamphlet
- occasional referral to a dietitian
- follow-up office visits with focus more on the medical problem than the weight problem.

But this approach nearly always fails, and those few who do lose weight typically regain it within a few weeks or months. The reasons for failure of weight loss programs are numerous and complex, but they share a unifying characteristic: lack of knowledge.

We need adequate knowledge of nutrition and how our bodies work to avoid wasting time, money, and energy on worthless weight-loss schemes. We must learn to easily identify weight-loss plans that are designed only to enrich the entrepreneur. We must learn to recognize scams that may jeopardize our physical and emotional health. Most importantly, knowledge is your key to successful long-term weight management. Given an adequate knowledge base, most people don't need to consult physicians, dietitians, or other advisers on weight loss.

Acquisition of that knowledge base, however, is not easy. Information and opinions are readily available from the Internet, books, television, magazines, newspaper articles, friends, acquaintances, health food store clerks, hearsay at the beauty salon, and advertisements for various weight-loss products. Much of this is worthwhile, much is worthless.

How do you separate the wheat from the chaff? The "doctor" in my doctor of medicine degree is based on the Latin word for "teacher." I'll share with you what your personal physician likely would teach you, if only he had the time. He would help you find the pearls of knowledge in a sea of complexity, confusion, contradiction, and quackery. My aim is to educate you so that you can seize control of your weight problem.

Although some of the information presented here is common knowledge, most of it is gleaned from my three decades of clinical experience with overweight patients and from my analysis of scientific literature generated by obesity researchers and clinicians.

The scientific literature is neither readily available nor understandable to the layperson. Furthermore, technical popularizers in the media tend to sensationalize preliminary research results. They may unwittingly promote fads since they lack the scientific training and clinical experience to recognize the real, but rare, breakthroughs. Having observed my patients' weight-loss efforts of every description, I know what works and what doesn't.

ACKNOWLEDGEMENTS

Sir Isaac Newton wrote in 1676: "If I have seen further, it is by standing on the shoulders of giants." He was acknowledging that his scientific success had been built upon the achievements of other scientists. While no one would ever mistake me for a Newton, I am similarly indebted to generations of scientists and physicians who have discovered and shared basic truths in the fields of nutrition, physiology, pathophysiology, and epidemiology. These are the foundations of this book.

I am grateful to Linda Kimmel, medical librarian, for her help acquiring the scientific literature, and to Scottsdale Healthcare for funding her position. I am obliged to innumerable dietitians and nutritionists who generously shared their knowledge with me. I am indebted to my patients, who helped me learn the art and science of medicine through the privilege of caring for them. Thanks to Art Chance for his participation years ago in our two-man think tank dedicated to improving health through exercise and nutrition.

Certain individuals have influenced my ideas about nutrition and fitness over the last few years in a positive way. A partial list (in no particular order) includes Monica Reinagel, Jimmy Moore, Regina Wilshire, Dave Dixon, Douglas Robb, Gary Taubes, Michael R. Eades, Robert C. Atkins, Laura Dolson, Lyle McDonald, Dr. J, Emily Deans, Tom Naughton, Beth Mazur, Sandy Szwarc, Travis Saunders, Peter Janiszewski, Richard David Feinman, Skyler Tanner, Darya Pino, Alex Hutchinson, K. Dunn Gifford, Yoni Freedhoff, Stephan Guyenet, Richard K. Bernstein, Arya M. Sharma, Dan Buettner, Conner Middelmann-Whitney, Jennifer Eloff, Eric Westman, Stephen Phinney, and Jeff Volek. I'm grateful to them for having stimulated my cerebral synapses. Any errors in this book are strictly mine, not theirs.

I thank my immediate family (Sunny, Dan, Brian, Casey, Paul, and Austin) for enduring my nutritional obsession, including recurrent dinner-table discussions of junk food, whole grains, calories, carbohydrates, and fiber. I am especially indebted to my wife for her role as steadfast supporter, sounding board, and Mediterranean chef. I love you, Sweet Pea. I thank God for enabling me to present this information to you. Any good that comes from it is from Him.

Introduction

"I've become my mother!" cried Janice as she studied her reflection in a full-length mirror on her 40th birthday. She had ballooned from 130 to 175 pounds (59 to 80 kg) over the last 15 years. Janice didn't think twice about her weight until after her first baby, Ashley, was born when Janice was 24. She gained 30 pounds (14 kg) during the pregnancy, but was down 15 pounds (6.8 kg) by the time she left the hospital. The other 15 pounds, which she called baby fat, hung around. During her teen years, Janice had been active in her school's marching band and regularly played softball. She jogged two or three miles a couple days per week, just to keep in shape for her beloved softball.

After Ashley was born, Janice still played softball, but couldn't find the time to jog. Her second child, James, was born two years after Ashley. Household life began to get hectic. Janice's husband was working 60-hour weeks at the tire store. Her mother, 40 pounds (18 kg) overweight, remarked how hard it was to chase Ashley around the house when she babysat. Janice decided to table softball until the kids were older.

Janice added another eight pounds of lingering baby fat while pregnant with James. She got a job at a call center six months after his birth. She sat most of the day, processing orders for various products. The family's evening meal, by necessity it seemed, was too often a sack of fast food she picked up on the way home. Janice didn't have the time or energy for exercise after cleaning, shopping, and laundering. She drank four cans of Dr. Pepper every day for the pleasure and a boost of energy.

The surgeon who removed Janice's gallstones at age 35 told her they were caused by her excess weight. She began to worry about other health effects and her lack of energy and stamina. Years after giving up softball, she tried jogging around the block just once and strained her right hamstring muscle. No more jogging for her, she decided.

Over the next five years, Janice tried many of the popular diets: low-fat, Atkins, cabbage soup, Nutri-System, Jenny Craig. They all worked great. For a while. She lost eight to 15 pounds (6.8 kg) , then lost her enthusiasm. Two months later she would be back up to her baseline weight, if not higher.

Since breast cancer runs in her family, Janice came to me for a routine physical and referral for a mammogram. At the end of our visit, she asked, almost as an afterthought, "Hey, doc, what can I do to get this weight off?" It was the end of my workday so we had time to chat. She shared her frustration with her prior weight-loss efforts. She told me her dream of fitting into some of her old clothes and wondered if her husband would ever again look at her the way he did when they were newlyweds. She mentioned the stress and time constraints of a two-teenager household, and how the teens would eat only two kinds of food: fast food and junk food. She told me how it hurt when she had to turn down the school's request to chaperone her son's four-mile nature hike with his class; she knew she just didn't have the stamina.

I shared with Janice my own frustration in dealing with my patients' medical problems that were caused or clearly aggravated by their excess weight. I saw hundreds of patients like Janice give their honest and best efforts to lose weight and keep it off, only to fail. Their medical problems were good for my business, but I longed for better outcomes for my patients. I had seen weight-loss methods of all kinds come and go, then come again. Surely, there had to be a better way. I vowed to review the situation comprehensively, to learn definitively what we should be eating and doing, and to share with Janice the results of my efforts. In these pages, you'll see what I discovered.

BASIC STATS

Sixty-six percent of adults in the United States are chubby, pudgy, portly, plump, rotund, stout, corpulent, or just plain fat. These adjectives fall somewhere on the spectrum from mildly overweight to morbidly obese. Overweight means having more adipose tissue (commonly known as fat) than is considered healthy or normal by historical standards. Obesity refers to the more extreme accumulations of fat. Of the 66% of us who are overweight or obese, about half are overweight and half are obese.

A healthy weight for a 5-foot, 4-inch person (163 cm) would be 108 to 145 pounds (49 to 66 kg) ; obesity starts at 175 pounds (79.5 kg). For someone 5-foot, 10-inches tall (178 cm), a healthy weight is 128 to 174 pounds (58 to 79 kg), with obesity starting at 208 pounds (94.5 kg).

Have you ever noticed in old photographs how everyone seemed so skinny, even gaunt? The pictures don't lie. In fact, photos tend to make us look heavier. Despite a barrage of popular media reports touting exercise, healthy lifestyles, and low-fat eating, the prevalence of adult obesity in the United States increased from 13% of us in 1960 to 34% in 2010. That's one in three.

And our children (ages 6–19) are learning by example: 19%—one in five kids—are now overweight, gradually rising over the last three decades.

About 30% of of men and 45% of women in the United States are dieting currently, either in pursuit of culturally ideal attractiveness or health and longevity.

WHAT CAUSES OVERWEIGHT?

It's complicated. I don't want to bore you with too many details, so here's a simplified explanation.

Overweight can be defined simply as excessive storage of energy in the form of fat. To some extent, it's the result of an imbalance between energy intake and energy expenditure. Energy intake is food. Energy expenditure is a combination of physical activity and metabolism.

Metabolism refers to the complex chemical and physical processes in our bodies that are necessary for the maintenance of life. In metabolism, some substances are broken down to produce energy for vital processes, such as breathing, blood circulation, and generation of body heat. The other side of metabolism is formation of vital substances and structures, as in tissue repair or blood production. When more energy (food) is put into the system than is necessary for metabolism and physical activity, the excess is stored as fat. That fat is available to produce energy just as the wax in a candle is burned to release its stored energy as light and heat. Indeed, some candles are made from fats (tallow).

The fine balance between energy intake and expenditure is influenced by numerous factors, including heredity, environment, psychology, and basic physiologic mechanisms.

INSULIN: THE FAT-BUILDING HORMONE

Insulin is a major hormone influencing fat accumulation. In response to eating carbohydrates (and proteins to a much lesser extent), the pancreas secretes insulin into the bloodstream to lower blood sugar levels that rise in response to digestion of carbohydrates. If we eat too many carbohydrates, the resulting blood sugar will be converted to fat tissue. Eating fewer carbohydrates lowers the amount of circulating insulin, which could help with weight management. More on this later.

HEREDITY

Studies documenting an association between heredity and obesity have lead to unnecessary discouragement of dieters. If your genes totally determine your degree of fatness, it would indeed be a waste of time fighting heredity. Accept your fate and pig out! But genes are only a piece of the puzzle. Note that Japanese-American men living in Hawaii and California are 15 pounds (6.8 kg) heavier and two to three times more likely to become obese than are their counterparts remaining in Japan. Furthermore, the prevalence of obesity in the United States has doubled since 1900. These data speak more in favor of environmental and cultural influences since the gene pool does not change nearly that fast.

AGING

In the United States, both men and women tend to gain excess fat weight from early adulthood to middle age, with body weight peaking around age 50 or 60. Doubtless, we tend to be less physically active as we get older, and therefore "burn" fewer calories (units of energy). It's also true that the rate of metabolism slows by 2% per decade in adulthood. If food intake doesn't diminish comparably, weight gain results. One-third of us are able to buck the weight gain trend.

ANCESTRY AND THE THRIFTY GENE HYPOTHESIS

Throughout most of human history, mere survival required a great expenditure of energy in the form of physical activity. Our forebears struggled to find and collect food, build shelter, and make clothing. Firewood for heat, cooking, and light was gathered piece by piece. Potable water was not available at simply the flick of a wrist.

In prehistoric days, abundant food was available sporadically and seasonally, if at all. Lacking refrigeration or other effective means of food storage, our ancestors gorged when they had the chance. Their goal was storage of food energy in the one place available to all: fat tissue. Those who could store more energy (fat) were more likely to survive the hardscrabble times when food was scarce due to poor weather, wildfires, disease, and competition. Survivors had genes that facilitated fat storage. For better or worse, they passed these genes down to us.

With the advent of the Neolithic Agricultural Revolution some 10,000 years ago, we became less dependent on the whims of nature. Crop cultivation yielded a steadier and larger supply of food while requiring less work. A few individuals, now with a bit of free time and excess energy, began the development of the arts, philosophy, music, science, and technology.

The Industrial Revolution of the late 18th century then freed the rest of us (in the developed world) from the constant, energy-draining struggle for mere survival. Scientific and technological advances afforded us the basic necessities of life with less physical labor. In 1900, well over two-thirds of the American work force was in farming; today fewer than 2% of us farm. Individuals can now expend yet more effort on intellectual pursuits, such as expansion of our knowledge base and further technological advances. We even have the time and energy for stamp collecting, surfing, bird-watching, fiddling, TV watching, and other such frivolities.

Whereas our ancestors spent untold hours and energy gathering fruit and berries or hunting game, we have labor-saving devices that wash our dishes and change our TV channel for us. Imagine how much more energy we would expend if not for refrigeration, plumbing, electricity, cars, computers, and telephones! As more machines and technology do our work, we require less food energy (calories). In reality, Americans eat more calories than we did 30 years ago.

In a nutshell, our increasingly prevalent overweight problem stems from a biological predisposition to store excess energy as fat, coupled with our sedentary lifestyles and abundant food. Compared to our Paleolithic ancestors, we have incredible access to grains, concentrated sugars, and vegetable or seed oils (such as corn and soybean oil).

If we just look at the last 100 years, we find our diets in the U.S. have changed dramatically. For example, refined sugar consumption in the U.S. was 11 lb (5 kg) in the 1830s, rising to 155 lb (70 kg) by 2000. Over the last 30 years in the U.S., consumption of sugar-sweetened beverages has increased from 3.9% of total calories to 9.2%. In that same time span, the percentage of overweight or obese American adults increased from 47% to 66%. The obesity percentage alone rose from 15 to 34% of adults.

Furthermore, soybean oil consumption increased from essentially zero a century ago to 7.4% of total calories today. Check the ingredients on processed food labels and there's a good chance you'll find soybean oil.

A RADICAL THEORY OF OBESITY FROM GARY TAUBES

At the start of my medical career three decades ago, many of my overweight patients were convinced they had a hormone problem causing the weight gain. I carefully explained that a hormone is rarely to blame. As it turns out, I may have been wrong. The hormone is insulin.

Science writer Gary Taubes has popularized what I'll call the "carbohydrate/insulin theory of obesity" in his 2007 masterpiece, *Good Calories, Bad Calories*. For details, the average consumer is better off reading his 2011 book, *Why We Get Fat*.

Mr. Taubes says, "We don't get fat because we overeat; we overeat because we're getting fat." Read that again and let it sink in. We need to think of obesity, says Taubes, as a disorder of excess fat accumulation, then ask why the fat tissue isn't regulated properly. A limited number of hormones and enzymes regulate fat storage; what's the problem with them?

Mr. Taubes makes a great effort to convince us the old "energy balance equation" doesn't apply to fat storage. You remember the equation: eat too many calories and you get fat, or fail to burn up enough calories with metabolism and exercise, and you get fat. To lose fat, eat less and exercise more. He prefers to call this the "calories-in/calories-out" theory. He admits it has at least a little validity. Problem is, the theory seems to have an awfully high failure rate when applied to weight management over the long run. We've operated under that theory for the last half century, but keep getting fatter and fatter. So the theory must be wrong on the face of it, right? Is there a better one?

Here is Taubes' explanation. The hormone in charge of fat storage is insulin; it works to make us fatter, building fat tissue. If you've got too much fat, you must have too much insulin action. And what drives insulin secretion from your pancreas? Dietary carbohydrates, especially refined carbs such as sugars, flour, cereal grains, starchy vegetables (e.g., corn, beans, rice, potatoes), and liquid carbohydrates. These are the "fattening carbs." Dozens of enzymes and hormones are at play either depositing fat into tissue, or mobilizing the fat to be used as energy. It's an active process going on continuously. Any regulatory derangement that favors fat accumulation will CAUSE gluttony (overeating) or sloth (inactivity). So it's not your fault.

If Taubes Is Right, How Do We Lose Excess Fat?

Cut back on carb consumption to lower your fat-producing insulin levels, and you turn fat accumulation into fat mobilization. Especially avoid the "fattening carbs."

Before you write off Taubes as a fly-by-night crackpot, be aware that he's received three Science-in-Society Journalism Awards from the National Association of Science Writers. He's a respected, professional science writer. Having read two of his books, it's clear to me he's very intelligent. If he's got a hidden agenda, it's well hidden.

One example illustrates how hormones control growth of tissues, including fat tissue. Consider the transformation of a skinny 11-year-old girl into a voluptuous woman of 18. Various hormones make her grow and accumulate fat in the places we now see curves. The hormones make her eat more, and they control the final product. The girl has no choice. Same with our adult fat tissue, but with different hormones. If some derangement is making us grow fatter, it's going to make us more sedentary (so more energy can be diverted to fat tissue) or make us overeat, or both. We can't fight it. At not least very well, as you can readily appreciate if look at the people around you at any American shopping mall.

If cutting carbohydrate consumption is so critical for long-term weight control, why is it that so many different diets—with no focus on carb restriction—seem to work, if only for the short run? Taubes suggests it's because nearly all diets reduce carbohydrate consumption to some degree, including the fattening carbs. If you reduce your total daily calories by 500, for example, many of those calories will be from carbohydrates. Simply deciding to "eat healthy" works for some people: stopping soda pop, candy bars, cookies, desserts, beer, etc. That cuts a lot of fattening carbs right there.

Losing excess weight or controlling weight by avoiding carbohydrates was the conventional wisdom prior to 1960, as documented by Mr. Taubes. Low-carb diets for obesity date back almost 200 years. The author attributes many of his ideas to German internist Gustav von Bergmann (1908).

Taubes rejects the calories-in/calories-out theory of overweight that hasn't done a very good job for us over the last 40 years. Taubes's alternative ideas deserve serious consideration.

STRAIGHT UP, DOC . . . WHY AM I FAT?

Remember that insulin is the major fat-building hormone, and carbohydrates are the main cause of insulin release from the pancreas. Refined starches and concentrated sugars in particular raise insulin output. Overweight in advanced countries is usually caused by excessive consumption of these fattening carbohydrates.

A LOOK AHEAD

Recall that overweight results from an imbalance between energy intake and energy expenditure. You must overcome this imbalance if you are to lose weight.

By the time you finish this book, you'll have the facts and motivation you need to lose your excess weight and keep it under control for the long run. We'll briefly review physiology and nutrition, then explore the consequences of obesity and the benefits of exercise in more depth. Only then will you be ready for my eating plan for successful weight loss. Finally, I'll tell you how to be successful at the most troublesome, frustrating, and mysterious area of weight control: long-term maintenance of weight loss.

KEY POINTS

- 66% of U.S. adults are overweight or obese.
- Fat is stored energy.
- We have a biological predisposition to store excess energy (calories) as fat. Sedentary lifestyles and abundant food contribute to fat storage.
- Insulin is the primary fat storage hormone.
- Overweight in advanced countries is usually caused by excessive consumption of fattening carbohydrates such as refined starches and concentrated sugars.
- Gary Taubes' "carbohydrate/insulin theory of obesity" is a major advancement in current thinking about the cause of overweight.

1

Why We Eat
and What Happens Next

"Would you like fries with that?" the clerk asked Tom after he ordered a Big Mac, apple pie, and chocolate shake at the drive-thru. He was already salivating. "Sure, why not?" Tom didn't realize, or care, that he had just ordered 1,770 calories, which is about what many people eat in an entire day. Tom eats three meals a day. It sure tasted good.

Tom grew up in a small Texas town. At age 17 he was 6-feet, 2-inches (188 cm) tall and large enough to help take his high school football team to the state championship playoff his junior and senior years. Football reigned supreme on Friday nights back in those days, not only for Tom, but the entire town. With weightlifting and football practice, Tom was exercising about three hours on most days and eating 5,000 to 6,000 calories. He didn't call it exercise, it was just who he was. He remembers often washing down an apple pie with a quart of milk in one sitting. Yes, the whole pie.

Like his father, Tom was a meat-and-potatoes kind of guy who ignored most fruits and vegetables. That was rabbit food. His favorite meal was slow-cooked barbecue brisket, potato salad, and baked beans flavored with brown sugar and bacon. Tom's wife, Barbara, knew that the men in his family were prone to overweight, heart attacks, high blood pressure, and high cholesterol. Tom stubbornly resisted her gentle pressure to eat healthier, whatever that meant. Eating was about enjoyment, in his mind, not about what his body needed.

Tom was a passable student and earned a football scholarship at a Texas college. A severe knee injury at the end of his sophomore season put the kibosh on his dreams of a pro football career and sidelined him for a good year while healing. He had always loved working with his hands, so he dropped out of college to become a full-time carpenter. His bosses at the construction company eventually rewarded his management skills by making him a supervisor. After that, he did less physical labor, but worked more hours. In his 30s, Tom still enjoyed the Friday night football games. But now he was sitting in the stands sipping sodas and chowing down on corn-dogs. He wasn't exercising three hours a day any-more, but he could still finish off a whole pie in a day. His only exercise was an occasional trip to the park to play catch with his young son.

Tom's father had his first heart attack at age 59, when Tom was 37. Dad had seemed the picture of health, except for the spare tire around his middle. Reality assaulted Tom with the fact that Dad might not always be around. Tom even thought about changing some of his own health habits. He heard all about the diet and lifestyle changes recommended by his father's doctors. Barbara made sure of that! But Dad recovered and Tom put health concerns on the back burner.

Six months later, Tom started having chest pains right behind the breastbone. His first thought was, "Oh, no! Is this what a heart attack feels like?" He couldn't have a heart attack at age 37, could he? Typical for a man, Tom ignored it as best he could. The first pains resolved spontaneously. The later pains seemed to improve with Maalox or Tylenol. But the pains got worse and more frequent. It was getting harder to hide it from Barbara.

During a particularly bad spell, he broke into a cold sweat as his heart palpitated. Realizing how bad off he was, he wondered if he would be around to see his son grow up. That's when he admitted he better get some professional help and a life insurance policy. Calling 911 was definitely the right thing to do. He let Barbara make the call, then he was admitted to my service at the hospital.

Tom was lucky. Tests showed he was only suffering from an unusually bad case of heartburn; stomach acid was irritating his esophagus. We could manage that condition with medication and diet changes, but his eating habits were sending him a warning. I shared with him my sense that he was headed toward an early heart attack, like his father. His eat-whatever-tastes-good diet, high blood pressure (154/100 mm/Hg)), high cholesterol (250 mg/dl or 6.5 mmol/l), high triglycerides (310 mg/dl or 3.5 mmol/l), sedentary ways, and his weight all added up to an unhealthy lifestyle. His "game weight" at age 20 was 220 pounds (100kg), all muscle and bone. Now he was 308 pounds (140 kg), with much less muscle. Tom's encounter with his own mortality accomplished what his wife's health-conscious exhortations could not. He was now ready to make major lifestyle changes, and asked for my guidance.

PHYSIOLOGY, NUTRITION, AND WEIGHT LOSS

If you have absolutely no interest in science or how your body runs, skip the rest of this chapter.

To lose your excess fat safely and permanently, you must understand how you acquired it in the first place and how fat tissue fits in with other components of your body. We need to review some basic principles of physiology and nutrition.

Physiology is the branch of biology dealing with the functions and vital processes of organisms or their parts and organs. Nutrients are substances in food that are used in the body to provide energy and structural materials, and to regulate the growth, maintenance, and repair of the body's tissues. Nutrition as a science is the study of nutrients in foods and of the body's handling of them in processes necessary for life, growth, and optimal health.

The commercial success of worthless weight-loss scams is testament that many people are relatively ignorant of nutrition and physiology. Some have forgotten what they once learned. Others are subject to wishful thinking or delusion. Many want to believe that weight loss is easy, that a session with a hypnotist will do the trick, that a vitamin and herb mix will "melt away the fat," that weight-loss pills alone are a safe long-term solution, that they can eat anything they want if they are in the right program. But wishing does not make it so.

There are six major classes of substances (called nutrients) that the body uses for growth, maintenance, and repair of tissues. They are water, fat, protein, carbohydrates, vitamins, and minerals.

A healthy 140 pound (64 kg) body contains about 85 pounds (39 kg) of water and 25 pounds (11 kg) of fat. The remaining 30 pounds (14 kg) are mostly protein, carbohydrate, and the bone minerals: calcium and phosphorus. All other minerals and vitamins together weigh less than a pound (0.5 kg).

Your body can make some nutrients for itself. But there are at least 40 specific nutrients, each one essential for health, that you can obtain only from food. Eating the right foods is critical.

WATER

Without water, there is no life as we know it. The sum of chemical and physical processes necessary for the maintenance of life is called metabolism. Nearly all these processes occur in, or are dependent on, water. Life is a myriad of chemical reactions mostly occurring inside cells. Cells are the smallest living structural units capable of independent functioning. Millions of cells of different types are joined together to form our various tissues and organs. In addition to participating in many chemical reactions, water transports various vital materials (such as vitamins, minerals, sugar, amino acids) within and between cells. Water carries waste products away from cells.

A healthy body is 55–60% water. On average, we lose three to four cups (800 ml) of water per day through sweating and breathing (water vapor). Also, the kidneys must produce at minimum two cups

(480 ml) of urine daily to carry away waste products. We must replace these obligatory water losses. Water balance is carefully regulated by interactions between the brain (hypothalamus, pituitary), kidneys, adrenal glands, mouth, and stomach.

Water is so important that we can only live a couple weeks without it.

FAT

For too long, dietary fat has been demonized as bad for us. In fact, it has many wonderful attributes as a component of our diets and bodies. As a nutrient, it provides us with fat-soluble vitamins (A, D, E, and K), enhances food flavor, and provides building blocks for cell structures (e.g., cell membranes) and hormones. Moreover, dietary fat is a great source of inexpensive energy. As part of our bodies, fat provides insulation to conserve heat, provides shock absorption and cushioning (e.g., the buttocks), and stores huge amounts of energy. In the sphere of human relations, sufficient fat in the right places is essential to physical attractiveness.

TERMINOLOGY OF FATS

"Fat" can refer to all three types of lipids: triglycerides, sterols, and phospholipids. But usually fat refers to triglycerides, which make up 99% of stored body fat.

Triglycerides are composed of carbon, oxygen, and hydrogen atoms arranged as a molecule of glycerol with three fatty acids attached. A fatty acid is a chain of carbon atoms with attached hydrogens and an acid group at one end.

Carbon atoms must have four bonds with adjacent atoms. A fatty acid carrying the maximum possible number of hydrogen atoms is "saturated." Red meat typically is high in saturated fatty acids. If a couple of adjacent hydrogen atoms are missing, the two side-by-side carbon atoms in the chain form a double bond.

A fatty acid with one double bond and two hydrogen atoms missing is a "monounsaturated fatty acid," such as oleic acid. Olive oil has lots of monounsaturated fatty acids such as oleic acid.

A fatty acid with two or more carbon double bonds (and four or more missing hydrogens) is "polyunsaturated," such as linolenic or linoleic acid. Most vegetable oils fit this description.

Vegetable and fish oils have an abundance of polyunsaturated fats. Olive and canola oils are rich in monounsaturates. The tropical oils are an exception. Despite plant origins, coconut and palm oils are primarily saturated.

Food manufacturers can synthesize fats by adding hydrogen to the carbon-to-carbon double bonds in liquid vegetable oils. Food labels often refer to these artificial fats as hydrogenated or partially hydrogenated vegetable oils, trans fats, or trans-fatty acids. "Trans" refers to the altered three-dimensional configuration of the new molecule.

A triglyceride is formed when the acid ends of three fatty acids attach to glycerol. Triglycerides usually contain mixtures of fatty acids with variable carbon chain lengths and degrees of saturation. Fats and oils are overwhelmingly—95 percent—triglycerides.

There are two fatty acids that we need but our bodies cannot make: linoleic and linolenic acid. Nutritionists call these "essential fatty acids" since we must eat them for optimal nutrition and, indeed, for life. We can make other fatty acids by combining two-carbon fragments derived from carbohydrates (e.g., sugar), protein, and alcohol. The new fatty acids attach to glycerol, forming triglycerides which can be taken up by adipose cells. This is how excessive intake of non-fat nutrients, especially carbohydrates, leads to overweight.

In addition to triglycerides, there are two other types of lipids: sterols and phospholipids. Well-known sterols are cholesterol, vitamin D, sex hormones, bile acids, and cortisol. They share a basic structure of carbon, oxygen, and hydrogen arranged in multiple rings.

Sterols in food are a minor source of calories. Our bodies synthesize the sterols we need for metabolic processes. For example, the liver manufactures the cholesterol that becomes a major component of new cell walls. Over 90% of total body cholesterol is tied up in cell walls.

Phospholipids have a structure similar to triglycerides but contain a few atoms of phosphorus and nitrogen. They serve primarily as cell wall components.

DO DIETARY FATS CAUSE HEART DISEASE?

Until just recently, physicians thought that dietary fat and saturated fats in particular were a major cause of atherosclerosis, also known as hardening of the arteries. The hardening isn't so bad; the problem is that it's accompanied by obstructive plaque in the walls of arteries. The plaque impairs the flow of blood to vital tissues, and the plaque can rupture, allowing the sudden formation of a blood clot that stops all blood flow. Tissue downstream from the clot dies. So atherosclerosis is the cause of most heart attacks, strokes, and poor circulation. It also contributes to high blood pressure.

The American Heart Association in 1957 recommended that polyunsaturated fats replace saturated fats in an effort to reduce heart and vascular disease. U.S. public health recommendations in 1977 were to reduce fat intake to 30% of total calories to lower the risk of coronary heart disease (atherosclerosis of the heart arteries). Slowly, some fats were replaced mostly with carbohydrates, highly refined ones at that. This shift tends to raise blood triglycerides and lower HDL cholesterol levels, which may themselves contribute to atherosclerosis. Current recommendations are, essentially, to keep saturated fatty acid consumption as low as possible.

The latest scientific evidence, however, indicates that total dietary fat and saturated fat have little, if anything, to do with causing atherosclerosis, heart attacks, strokes, or poor circulation in most people. (For details, see Selected References at the end of the book.) In fact, replacing dietary fats with carbohydrates may have contributed significantly to the steady rise in overweight and obesity we've seen over the last forty years in the U.S.

Trans fats, however, are still thought to contribute to heart and vascular disease. Food manufacturers using these man-made fats continue to reduce utilization in response to public pressure and concern. A safe minimal level of consumption has never been established.

DIGESTION AND UTILIZATION OF FATS

After a meal, digestive juices inside the small intestine go to work on ingested fats (triglycerides), removing two or all three of the fatty acids from the glycerol molecule. The resulting pieces are absorbed by cells lining the small intestine, where they are reassembled into triglycerides. These new triglycerides are extruded into the bloodstream and circulate all over the body to be used either as an immediate source of energy or stored in fat tissue as a future energy supply. Fat cells pluck any excess triglycerides from blood and store them as a glob of fat.

Later, when other cells need fuel energy, fat cells break down the triglycerides and kick fatty acids and glycerol into the bloodstream. The energy-starved cells pick up these triglyceride fragments and break them down further in chemical reactions that ultimately yield carbon dioxide, water, and energy.

Thanks to fat stores, a person of average weight can survive up to two months of total starvation. A fatter person can survive even longer.

PROTEIN

Proteins are complex chains of amino acids that play vital roles:
- in growth, replacement, and repair of all tissues
- as enzymes regulating chemical processes
- as antibodies fighting infection
- in fluid balance
- in acid-base balance
- as hormones (e.g., insulin, thyroid

hormone)
- in blood clotting
- as an emergency energy source when carbohydrates and fats are limited.

Amino acids have a central carbon atom with four attachments: a hydrogen atom, an amino group, an acid group, and a variable side group or side chain. The 20 common amino acids are distinguished by their individual side groups.

Most proteins are composed of between 20 to several hundred amino acid building blocks linked together chain-like in a specific sequence. Chains of amino acids may also be linked together, often via sulfur atoms, to form even larger complex molecules. For instance, insulin consists of a specific sequence of 51 amino acids in two chains linked by sulfur bridges.

Food digestion breaks down dietary protein into its component amino acids, which we then use to make the proteins we need. If not available from the diet, our bodies can synthesize 11 of the 20 common amino acids.

But there are nine amino acids that we cannot make and must obtain from food. These are referred to as "essential amino acids." If not in the diet, the body will break down its own proteins to obtain these essential amino acids. Avoid this self-cannibalism by eating the right foods!

Formation of protein in a cell requires that all the needed amino acids be available simultaneously. Non-essential amino acids are pulled out of the circulating pool or manufactured right in the cell. But if the diet supplies too little of an essential amino acid, protein synthesis will be limited. Over time, the result is malnutrition.

A "complete protein" food contains all nine of the essential amino acids, in about the right proportions as humans require. Proteins in foods from animals—poultry, fish, meat, eggs, cheese, and milk—are generally complete. Eggs and milk contain particularly high-quality proteins.

Plant-derived foods provide less protein per unit of measure, and tend to be deficient in one or more essential amino acids. Soy protein, however, is complete and is sometimes used as a meat replacement. Vegetarians who exclude all animal-derived foods can receive all the amino acids they need if they eat a variety of legumes, grains, vegetables, nuts, and seeds (e.g., sunflower, sesame). The idea is to combine two or more foods so that the essential amino acids missing from one are supplied by the other.

For healthy adults, the protein Recommended Dietary Allowance is 0.8 grams per kilogram of appropriate body weight per day. This is about 50 grams for an average-sized person. As examples, a slice of bread has three grams of protein, a cup (240 ml) of milk has eight grams, a cup of beans has 13 grams, and three ounces (84 g) of meat has 21 grams of protein. We in the United States generally eat much more protein than needed.

CARBOHYDRATES

Carbohydrates mainly serve as a source of energy for us, providing about half of the energy in the standard American diet. The other half comes mostly from fat. Relatively little of our energy comes from protein.

There are essential amino acids (in proteins) and there are essential fatty acids (in fats): "essential" meaning our bodies cannot make them so we must eat them for life and health. There are no essential carbohydrates; we can make the ones we need.

Carbohydrates contain only carbon, oxygen, and hydrogen.

The most fundamental carbohydrate is a simple sugar called glucose. It's used as an energy source by all the cells in our body. It's like the gasoline needed to run a car, a car that's always running. Although we eat relatively little pure glucose, most dietary carbohydrates are converted during digestion to glucose, which is used as fuel. Any excess glucose not needed immediately for energy is converted to a storage form, called glycogen, for later use. We have the capacity to store only a half day's worth of energy in glycogen. Carbohydrates are converted to fat when eaten in excess of what we can use immediately as energy or store as glycogen.

The preceding paragraph is exceedingly important for anyone with an excess weight problem. Read it again.

Carbohydrates are composed of sugars. Basic sugar molecules contain six carbon atoms, twelve hydrogen atoms, and six oxygen atoms. The various atoms are arranged in simple structures to form the three most basic sugars: glucose, fructose, and galactose. These ring-like structures are called monosaccharides.

When a chemical reaction joins a pair of monosaccharides together, the result is a disaccharide. The one most familiar to you is sucrose, or table sugar.

Sucrose, lactose, and maltose are the three most important disaccharides. Each of them has a glucose ring molecule attached to a ring of fructose, galactose, or another glucose. Lactose is the major carbohydrate in milk, contributing up to 50 percent of its calories. The monosaccharides and disaccharides are "simple carbohydrates," also called sugars.

"Complex carbohydrates" are much larger molecules composed of straight or branched chains of linked monosaccharides, mostly glucose. The three important complex carbohydrates, also known as polysaccharides, are starch, glycogen, and fiber.

Starch is a storage form of energy in plants. Through photosynthesis, green plants use sunlight's energy to form carbohydrates from carbon dioxide and water. Carbohydrates not used as structural parts of the plant can be stored as glucose chains, i.e., starch. After planting, the starch in a grain of corn supplies energy to the seedling until it can capture sunlight's energy through its leaves. Starchy foods such as wheat, rice, potatoes, and legumes provide not only energy but potentially a wealth of vitamins, minerals, and other healthful substances if they are not removed by processing.

Glycogen is a storage form of energy in animals. It's composed of numerous glucose molecules tied together in highly branched chains. In contrast, starch chains in plants are unbranched or only occasionally branched. Glycogen and starch are otherwise so similar that glycogen is sometimes referred to as animal starch. One third of total body glycogen is in the liver, two thirds is in muscle tissue. Muscle is stingy, tending to hold onto glycogen-glucose for its own use. On the other hand, a major function of the liver is to rapidly breakdown glycogen and release glucose into the bloodstream whenever another tissue needs energy.

Fibers are mostly complex carbohydrates forming the structural parts of plants. Cellulose is a good example since it's the primary structural element of all plant cell walls and you're familiar with it as a component of paper. Human digestive enzymes cannot break down the types of bonds between fiber monosaccharide units. Fiber passes undigested through the small intestine, but bacteria in the large intestine partially digest it. This benefits the bacteria and we get a few short-chain fatty acids in the bargain.

Eating too much dietary fiber can cause intestinal discomfort and gas, may interfere with absorption of some nutrients (e.g., minerals), and may be so filling that they displace other necessary nutrients that we might have eaten if not full. That's not a big worry, though. Inadequate fiber intake is much more prevalent and may have adverse health consequences. The potential health benefits of high dietary fiber intake include:

- lower blood cholesterol
- improved blood glucose levels in diabetics
- improved weight control
- prevention of constipation, hemorrhoids, and diverticulosis

DIGESTION AND UTILIZATION OF CARBOHYDRATES

When you eat a baked potato or bowl of rice, chewing stimulates the salivary glands to secrete an enzyme that starts breaking down complex carbohydrates into smaller polysaccharides. The small intestine does the bulk of digestive work; chemical reactions governed by enzymes disassemble starches and disaccharide sugars down to mono-saccharide units (glucose, fructose, and galactose). Monosaccharides are absorbed into the blood and flow downstream to the liver, where fructose and galactose are converted to glucose.

At this point you have a hefty load of glucose in the liver and must "decide" what to do with it. There are only two choices: kick it back into the bloodstream for distribution to energy-hungry cells, or store it as energy to use later. If you're already overweight, you want to store it as glycogen instead of fat, or burn it up as an energy source right now.

One of the liver's major functions is to store glucose (as glycogen) and release it as needed. Cells need a constant energy supply and can get that energy from glucose or fat. Some tissues, most notably the brain and nerves, are almost entirely dependent on glucose as their energy source. Cells take glucose out of circulation and split it into smaller fragments, yielding energy, carbon dioxide, and water.

Even when cells use fat for energy they still need some glucose for the most efficient utilization of fat.

Our bodies have elaborate mechanisms for maintaining blood glucose at an optimal range (about 70–140 milligrams per deciliter or 3.9–7.8 mmol/l) so that cells, particularly in the brain and nerves, don't "run out of gas." Blood glucose falling too low triggers the breakdown of glycogen into glucose, which the liver pumps into the bloodstream.

Just how much glucose is circulating in our bloodstreams anyway? In a normal, healthy state, not much: about a teaspoon (5 ml).

While fat tissue stores enough energy to last for weeks, we can only store enough glycogen to last a matter of hours. When it is gone, the body can produce significant amounts of glucose only by disassembling proteins or fats.

Your body just isn't able to convert much fat into glucose. Remember that fats are triglycerides: three fatty acid chains attached to a small glycerol molecule. You can convert the glycerol into glucose, but glycerol is only 5% of the fat molecule. The fatty acids can be broken down through a process called fatty acid oxidation, producing energy, but not glucose. Our bodies can also make limited amounts of glucose from dietary protein or by breaking down our own body proteins.

So the glucose your body craves as immediate fuel usually comes from daily dietary carbohydrates, or from the limited glycogen stored in your body.

What happens if you drastically reduce your consumption of carbohydrates for days on end? Where do your cells get the energy needed to survive and thrive? It gets most of it from your body fat stores, which break down to fatty acids and glycerol. The fatty acids are metabolized (oxidized) to supply energy to most tissues. Glycerol and proteins provide the glucose needed by the brain and nerves.

This switch in energy metabolism from one based on carbohydrates to one based on fats is how, for example, people can live for a couple months without any food whatsoever. It also explains how we sleep through a long night and skip occasional meals without adverse effects.

The idea that we need to eat carbohydrates every few hours to keep our energy up is a myth.

Insulin and Carbohydrate Handling

The digestion of a meal containing carbohydrates causes blood sugar (glucose) levels to rise. In response, the pancreas gland secretes insulin into the bloodstream to keep sugar levels from rising too high. The insulin drives the excess sugar out of the blood, into our tissues. Once inside the tissues' cells, the glucose will be used as an immediate energy source or stored for later use. Excessive sugar is stored either as body fat or as glycogen in liver and muscle.

When we digest fats, we see very little direct effect on blood sugar levels. That's because fat contains almost no carbohydrate. In fact, when fats are eaten with high-carbohydrate foods, it tends to slow the rise and peak in blood sugar you'd see if you had eaten the carbohydrates alone.

Ingested protein can and does raise blood sugar, usually to a mild degree. As proteins are digested, our bodies can make sugar (glucose) out of the breakdown products. The healthy pancreas releases some insulin to keep the blood sugar from going too high.

In contrast to fats and proteins, carbohydrates in food cause significant—often dramatic—rises in blood sugar. Our pancreas, in turn, secretes higher amounts of insulin to prevent excessive elevation of blood glucose. Carbohydrates are easily digested and converted into blood sugar. The exception is fiber, which is indigestible and passes through us unchanged.

During the course of a day, the pancreas of a healthy person produces an average of 40 to 60 units of insulin. Half of that insulin is secreted in response to meals, the other half is steady state or "basal" insulin. The exact amount of insulin depends quite heavily on the amount and timing of carbohydrates eaten. Dietary protein has much less influence. A pancreas in a healthy person eating a very-low-carbohydrate diet will release substantially less than 50 units of insulin a day.

To summarize thus far: dietary carbohydrates are the major source of blood sugar for most people eating "normally." Carbohydrates are, in turn, the main cause for insulin release by the pancreas, to keep blood sugar levels in a safe, healthy range.

You've learned that insulin's main action is to lower blood sugar by transporting it into the cells of various tissues. But that's not all insulin does. It also 1) impairs breakdown of glycogen into glucose, 2) stimulates glycogen formation, 3) inhibits formation of new glucose molecules by the body, 4) promotes storage of triglycerides in fat cells (i.e., lipogenesis, fat accumulation), 5) promotes formation of fatty acids (triglyceride building blocks) by the liver, 6) inhibits breakdown of stored triglycerides, and 7) supports body protein production.

Insulin actions No.4 and No.5 are particularly problematic if you're trying to get rid of excess body fat. To paraphrase: insulin promotes storage of body fat and impairs breakdown of existing fat tissue. Not good if you want to get rid of excess fat. In that instance, wouldn't it make sense to try to reduce insulin release by the pancreas? You do that by cutting down on easily digestible carbohydrates like sugar-sweetened drinks and refined flours and starches. Or reduce total carbohydrate consumption. Or both.

VITAMINS

I vividly recall a patient of mine, a known alcoholic, who was brought to the emergency room by his wife because he was unable to walk without help. He was fine until a few days earlier when he noticed spells of double vision. I found him also to be confused and cross-eyed. He wasn't drunk. His prompt improvement after an infusion of a specific vitamin into his blood-stream confirmed my suspicion: he had a thiamine deficiency.

Vitamins are organic substances that are vitally necessary in small amounts for normal growth and activity of our bodies. All can be obtained naturally from food. We only need tiny amounts since they are not energy sources or tissue building blocks.

Thus far in nutritional science, 13 vitamins have been identified. They are divided into categories based on whether they dissolve in water or fat/oil.

The water-soluble vitamins are vitamin C, the B vitamins (thiamine (B1), riboflavin (B2), niacin (nicotinic acid), biotin, pantothenic acid, B6 (pyridoxine), folate (folic acid), and B12 (cobalamin).

The fat-soluble vitamins are A, D, E, and K.

Fat-soluble vitamins are stored in our fat tissue and are released to the other tissues as needed over weeks or months. Water-soluble vitamins generally cannot be stored; excess intake is flushed out quickly by the kidneys. The take-home point: we need to eat water-soluble vitamins almost every day.

Vitamin deficiency diseases are uncommon in the developed world, thanks to an abundance of various foods and food fortification with added vitamins (e.g., flour with folate, milk with vitamin D). In fact, disorders of vitamin overdose may be more common than deficiency. It's a different story in parts of the Third World. Vitamin A deficiency, for example, is a major nutritional problem in the developing world, contributing to childhood blindness and premature death from infections.

Each vitamin has a specific job description in the business of nutritional physiology. Vitamins typically assist the enzymes that govern all the chemical reactions that constitute life. Here's a sampler of vitamin functions:

- assist cell growth and multiplication (B vitamins)
- assist energy production (B vitamins)
- promote nerve growth and protection (B12)
- serve as anti-oxidants that interfere with free radicals, thereby preventing damage to cell structures and alteration of normal cell functions (C, E)
- help with formation of collagen, the major structural protein in connective tissue
- help with formation of thyroid hormone and epinephrine
- promote healthy bones (A, D, K)
- essential to vision (A)
- help with formation of proteins that are responsible for blood clotting (K).

Lack of a single vitamin can kill you. Until the mid-18th century, sailors on long voyages commonly suffered that fate. Vegetables and fruits deteriorated more rapidly than other food provisions, so they were eaten early in the voyage. Later on, sailors predictably developed easy bruising, bleeding gums, poor wound healing, joint pains, and progressive weakness. Many eventually died from the disease scurvy. Suspecting a nutritional deficiency as the cause, a British physician in 1747 discovered that lime juice prevented the illness. To this day, "limey" is a slang term for a British sailor. Scientists later identified the single vital substance in lime juice as vitamin C.

Although vitamins are individually necessary for life, it is important to know that they work in concert with each other and with the other nutrients. Like the individual musicians in an orchestra, all the vitamins must be present and balanced to produce a beautiful work of art.

Full-blown vitamin deficiencies are rare in developed Western cultures. It is certainly possible, yet difficult to prove, that many people have mild vitamin (and mineral) deficiencies causing fatigue, malaise, weakness, lethargy, dizziness, or other nonspecific symptoms. Other causes are usually responsible. But without a doubt, such symptoms sometimes improve when a poor diet is altered to include a greater amount and variety of vitamins and minerals.

Several professional nutrition associations have recommended that healthy, non-pregnant adults not use vitamin supplements ordinarily. There are well-defined important exceptions to the general rule, so you should not stop a supplement recommended by your physician or registered dietitian. Most nutrition professionals recommend you obtain all your vitamins and other nutrients from a variety of whole foods: fruits, vegetables, grains, legumes, nuts, dairy products, fish, meat, poultry, and eggs.

To be absolutely certain you are getting all your necessary vitamins, I recommend you take a multivitamin when you start the Advanced or Ketogenic Mediterranean Diet.

MINERALS

Like the preceding nutrients we have reviewed, minerals are necessary for life. "Organic" nutrients are primarily based on the carbon atom and include fats, proteins, carbohydrates, and vitamins. In contrast, minerals are not based on carbon. They are inorganic elements that can carry an electrical charge when dissolved in water.

Our major minerals, in order of decreasing amounts in the body, are calcium, phosphorus, potassium, sulfur, sodium, chloride, and magnesium. The levels of all the minerals are tightly controlled by the kidneys, gastrointestinal tract, cell walls, hormones, and certain vitamins. Major minerals are most notable for their roles in:

- fluid balance, both inside and outside of cells
- regulation of acid-base balance
- structure of skeleton and teeth
- proper nerve and muscle function.

The average person has 2.5 pounds (1.1 kg) of calcium, 99% of which is in bones and teeth, contributing to structural integrity of the body. Calcium is also essential for blood clotting and function of muscles and nerves.

Phosphorus (1.5 pounds or 0.7 kg) is also a major component of bones and teeth. It is also important in acid-base balance, energy metabolism (e.g., adenosine triphosphate), cell walls (e.g., phospholipids), and in DNA-RNA.

Fluid balance is particularly dependent on sodium, chloride, and potassium.

Magnesium plays important roles in muscle and nerve function, protein production, energy metabolism, and bone mineralization.

Sulfur helps determine the shape of many protein molecules (e.g., insulin) and is a component of some vitamins and amino acids.

Minerals present in much smaller amounts, while still necessary for life, are called trace minerals. All together, our trace minerals might fill a couple thimbles.

It's impossible to discuss the functions of trace minerals without mentioning enzymes since they are linked intimately. Metabolism is the total of all chemical reactions that go on in living cells. In a chemical reaction, a substance is broken down, or is combined with other substances, or interchanges parts with other substances. In any case, the original substance is changed. Enzymes are special proteins that serve as catalysts for chemical reactions, speeding them up, without themselves being altered in the process. Trace minerals often serve as cofactors to enzymes, meaning that a specific mineral must be associated with a specific enzyme before the enzyme will work.

The most important trace minerals are iron, manganese, copper, iodide, selenium, zinc, fluoride, chromium, molybdenum, arsenic, nickel, silicon, and boron.

Iron is well-known for its role in blood formation. Red blood cells are loaded with hemoglobin, a protein that carries oxygen and releases it in the tissues where needed. The production and function of hemoglobin are both dependent on adequate iron intake. Eighty percent of the body's iron is in hemoglobin. Iron is found in many enzymes and works with the enzymes that produce energy in every cell. Iron deficiency is the most common trace mineral deficiency in the world.

Iodide is a key component of thyroid hormone, which regulates metabolic rate, body temperature, nerve and muscle function, reproduction, and heart function. Thanks to iodization of salt in developed countries, iodine deficiency is now rare.

Chromium is active in carbohydrate and lipid metabolism. It participates in the action of insulin. Diets low in chromium seem to cause abnormal elevations of blood sugar (glucose).

Copper is a constituent of enzymes affecting multiple diverse chemical reactions. It is a key factor in production of hemoglobin.

Zinc also is a cofactor to a multitude of enzymes all over the body. I mention zinc mainly to illustrate that an unbalanced intake of nutrients can be harmful. Excessive zinc intake, as in a nutritional supplement, can decrease the absorption of copper from the intestinal tract. Although rare, this can lead to copper-deficiency anemia.

Now close your book and take out a clean sheet of paper and a pencil for a pop quiz.

Don't sweat it! You won't have to remember all this stuff to be successful with the Advanced Mediterranean Diet. We've reviewed the basic attributes of various nutrients by themselves. Now let's tie it all together.

THE BIG PICTURE

Every single bite of food you swallow will be used in one or more of three possible ways:
1. for immediate energy
2. stored as energy (as fat or glycogen)
3. growth, maintenance, or repair of tissues.

While maintenance and repair of tissues are important to all of us, growth is a major issue in children, adolescents, and pregnant women. Proteins are the primary ingredient for growth and tissue maintenance and repair. That's why we eat proteins. They are not major energy-yielding nutrients.

We obtain energy from the chemical bonds between atoms in nutrients. The main energy-yielding nutrients are carbohydrates and fats. Chemical reactions break the bonds between the atoms, releasing the energy stored in the bonds. Much more energy can be released when oxygen is used in energy-producing chemical reactions. We huff and puff during exercise so we can pick up and deliver more oxygen to working muscle cells. Heavy breathing also blows off the carbon dioxide that is a byproduct of energy metabolism.

We must have energy to fuel two fundamental life processes: 1) basal metabolism, and 2) physical activity.

BASAL METABOLIC RATE

Basal metabolism refers to all the physiologic processes and chemical reactions that keep us alive in a resting state. These include maintenance of body temperature, breathing, continuous blood production, routine maintenance of healthy tissues, 100,000 heartbeats daily, etc. About 70% of our energy intake is used just for basal metabolism. Basal metabolic rate (BMR) is the rate at which the body uses energy (calories) for life-maintaining activities while lying down in a comfortable room with an empty stomach. These processes may require 1,200 to 1,500 calories per day for an average person, although there is large variability.

While heredity has a significant effect on BMR, a number of other conditions also affect it, and some are under our control. Factors that increase BMR include youth, tall and thin physique, growth (including pregnancy), higher muscle mass, stress, hot or cold environment, and overactive thyroid. Factors that decrease BMR include aging, excess fat tissue, fasting, starvation, malnutrition, and underactive thyroid.

There's no quick, easy, safe way to increase basal metabolic rate. If there were, losing excess weight would be a cinch. We would simply rev up our metabolism and fuel it with the energy stored in fat.

ENERGY EXPENDITURE

In addition to basal metabolism, the other major component of energy expenditure has the potential to convert our excess fat to actual energy. That component is physical activity. In theory, it sounds easy to increase exercise levels and burn off excess fat. In reality, it's difficult and usually doesn't make a major contribution to loss of excess weight. It seems to work on The Biggest Loser TV show. But how realistic is that situation for the average person? Not very.

Why doesn't exercise work better? It's not entirely clear, but a number of issues undoubtedly come into play. Exercise may stimulate appetite and lead to higher food consumption. It may be too hard to stick with a rigorous program. In terms of weight management, it's much easier to just skip the candy bar than to jog on a treadmill for 45 minutes to burn off the calories in the candy.

Muscles move us about by contracting, which requires energy. Heart rate and breathing rate increase above basal rates to supply muscles with oxygen and nutrients, and remove waste byproducts. On average, we use 20 to 30% of our energy on physical activity. An athlete in a vigorous training program may use 60 to 70% of his energy for exercise and only 30 to 40% for basal metabolism.

Physical activity in adulthood tends to decrease an average of 3% per decade, likely contributing to weight gain.

ENERGY PRODUCTION

Food is composed of various atoms bonded together. These bonds contain energy that is released when the bonds are broken by digestive and metabolic processes. The familiar calorie is a measurement of the energy-producing potential contained in food.

Fat is an excellent source of calories, with nine calories per gram. (A gram is about the weight of an aspirin tablet.) Carbohydrate and protein have four calories per gram. Alcohol can also provide energy: seven calories per gram. Most foods are a combination of carbohydrate, protein, fat, vitamins, and minerals. Carbohydrates and fats are our major sources of energy.

Carbohydrates are broken down to glucose, which is used as an immediate energy source, or stored in limited amounts as glycogen. The body keeps enough glycogen to fuel us only for a matter of hours. Beyond that, excess carbohydrates are converted to fat. Fat can be broken down later, when its stored energy is needed.

Dietary fat is digested into fatty acids, which are used as an immediate energy supply. If their energy is not needed, fatty acids are reunited with glycerol and stored as fat. Breakdown of fats does yield small amounts of glucose.

Proteins in food are broken down to their component amino acids, which can be 1) used as an immediate energy supply (often by conversion to glucose), 2) converted to triglycerides and stored as fat, or 3) used to assemble new proteins the body needs. Our bodies prefer to use the amino acids in food to construct new proteins we need for growth, repair, and maintenance of body tissues.

Carbohydrates (via glucose) are the best source of immediate energy. Fats are the next best source. We can train our bodies to use fats rather than carbohydrates as the primary energy source. When carbohydrates and fats are not available, the body will use amino acids for energy, even if it has to break down its own proteins to get amino acids for conversion to glucose. Remember that the brain and nerves must have glucose. If proteins are consumed in excess of the body's need for amino acids, they are converted into an immediate energy supply (glucose) or to fat. Excess amino acids cannot be stored for use later. On the other hand, if we don't eat enough protein, our body proteins break down to supply essential amino acids needed more urgently elsewhere in the body. Over time, this leads to muscle wasting.

BALANCED NUTRITON

All the aforementioned chemical reactions require the presence and proper balance of all the various nutrients, including vitamins and minerals. As an example, consider the major blood protein called hemoglobin. Iron is a key component of this large molecule, although it is primarily composed of amino acids derived from protein you eat. Let's say you eat plenty of protein. But if you don't ingest enough iron, you won't be able to make adequate amounts of hemoglobin. You'll be anemic; you won't have enough blood and will feel tired all the time.

ENERGY BALANCE EQUATION

Since you're interested in losing weight, you must never forget that the energy content of everything you eat will either be used as energy within hours, or stored as fat or glycogen.

Nearly all the energy we ingest as food is used within hours to fuel basal metabolism or physical activity. This is true even for grossly obese people. If your weight is stable over time, you are in "energy balance," even if you weigh 350 pounds (159 kg). You're burning up as many calories as you take in. If you've gradually gained 10 pounds (4.5 kg) over the last two years, your energy equation is slightly out of balance: you've eaten more energy than your body needed, and the excess is stored in your adipose tissue. If you wish to lose weight, you must tip the balance in the other direction, converting fat into the energy your body needs. There are only three ways to do this: 1) eat less food, 2) increase your basal metabolic rate, or 3) increase your physical activity.

The living human organism is an incredibly complex system. In terms of fundamental understanding of life, scientists have only scratched the surface. But they've discovered enough details so that you can become and stay healthy for as long as possible. Such knowledge is useless to you unless applied.

KEY POINTS

- Metabolism is the sum of chemical and physical processes necessary for the maintenance of life.
- Good health requires the proper mix of nutrients: water, fat, protein, carbohydrates, vitamins, and minerals.
- Nine of the amino acids we need can be obtained only from proper food choices, so they are essential.
- The two essential fatty acids, linoleic and linolenic, can only be obtained through correct food choices.
- There are no "essential carbohydrates" that we must obtain from food.
- Vitamins are organic substances that are vitally necessary in small amounts for normal growth and activity. Lack of a single vitamin can kill you.
- We must eat water-soluble vitamins frequently since we cannot store them in our bodies as we do fat-soluble vitamins.

55

- Every single bite of food you swallow will be used in one of three ways: 1) for immediate energy, 2) for growth, maintenance, or repair of tissues, or 3) or stored as energy in the form of glycogen or fat.
- The two determinants of our fuel requirements are basal metabolism and physical activity.
- If you wish to lose weight, there are only three possible ways: 1) eat less, 2) increase your basal metabolic rate, or 3) increase your physical activity.

2
I'm Fat. So What?

"I'm sorry, Matt, but we gave the promotion to Carlos," said Matt's boss. "You're a great employee and we don't want to lose you, but we have to do what's best for the company. I'm glad to give you a 3% raise. Thanks for your loyal service."

Matt was a graphic designer for an advertising agency. He had been with the company for four years. The quality of his work couldn't be beat. He was funny and likable. His attendance and timeliness were impeccable. He enjoyed brainstorming with the other designers if they needed help meeting their deadlines, even if he had to stay late. Matt had been awarded "Employee of the Year" after his third year with the agency. He was the "go-to guy" for many of the account executives when they needed fresh ideas.

Carlos, on the other hand, had been with the firm for only two years. The quality of his work was OK, but it was clear he would never set the advertising world on fire. He always clocked out at five o'clock sharp. As might be expected in an advertising firm, image was everything. The company owners and most of the bosses were fitness buffs. Several were known to have had cosmetic surgery. Carlos entertained the bosses and office ladies with his tales of rock climbing and competitive cycling. To top it off, Carlos was a dead ringer for Antonio Banderas.

The promotion involved the agency's first satellite office on the other side of the city. They needed a chief designer who would have creative control and supervise three other designers. The position would have almost doubled Matt's salary. Matt couldn't help but wonder if his weight, 325 pounds (148 kg), was the reason he was passed over. He didn't fit the corporate image of sleek and fit. He recalled the time a year previously his office chair collapsed under him. Everyone heard the commotion and rushed over. Was it his weight, or a defective chair that would have dumped anyone? His co-workers were too kind to speculate out loud. But, even now, Matt felt a rush of anxiety just thinking about the incident.

Matt had always been fat, even in childhood. He didn't know why. His parents were a little over-weight, about like everyone else. He was too heavy in childhood to do well in sports, so he developed other interests and talents. He dated girls occasionally, but even less after he graduated from college. Women didn't seem too interested in him romantically. Many just wanted to be friends.

Matt was sedentary. Given the choice of walking up a flight of stairs or taking the elevator, he always took the lift. He wondered, periodically, if he could slim down by exercising. His friends invited him to participate in their team sports, but he turned them down, fearing that he would drag down the team's performance with his weight and lack of physical fitness. He tried walking outside regularly, even though that was quite difficult after he passed 275 pounds (125 kg). It also bored him to tears. Five months out of the year it was too hot and humid even for walking. Tennis was hard on his ankles. His weight exceeded the limit for a rowing shell. He enjoyed bocce, but couldn't find other players. Golf was too expensive and time-consuming. Miniature golf didn't burn many calories. He was in a bowling league, but realized it wasn't much of a workout. Bicycling gave him a rash "down there."

Recently, Matt had been sleeping poorly at night and was sleepy during the day. He didn't feel well-rested when he woke up in the morning. His house-mate noted that Matt snored loudly and tossed and turned all night long, although he seemed to be asleep. He even seemed to stop breathing for brief spells while asleep. Matt figured his sagging mattress was the problem, so he replaced it even though he was only four years into the 10-year warranty. It didn't help. 28-year-old Matt came to see me for help with daytime sleepiness.

PSYCHOSOCIAL ASPECTS

Nobody ever says anything good about being over-weight, but there are advantages. By putting stress on the bones, obesity keeps them strong and prevents osteoporosis. Fat tissue fills in wrinkles, making the skin look younger. Abundant fat stores serve as insulation, conserving body heat, and allow you to survive longer during periods of starvation. Since

59

many of us currently don't consider excessive weight to be physically attractive, obesity can help you avoid unwanted sexual advances. Physical attractiveness is associated with higher income, but also lower scores on IQ tests and, in women, with being less satisfied with life in middle age. Being overweight and unconcerned about the consequences lets you eat all the delicious food you can get your lips on.

Actually, there is an organization that says good things about being overweight: the National Association to Advance Fat Acceptance. Founded in 1969, NAAFA is "dedicated to protecting the rights and improving the quality of life for fat people. NAAFA works to eliminate discrimination based on body size and provide fat people with the tools for self-empowerment through advocacy, public education, and support."

But there's another side to this coin. Are the advantages of fatness worth the teasing, the loss of mobility, the nagging from relatives and friends, the social isolation? Are they worth the extra wear and tear on furniture and clothing, the embarrassment of not fitting in the seat of an airplane or theater, the feelings of failure and inferiority, the adverse discrimination in social and job settings? I'm neither condoning nor justifying any of these situations; they are simply reality for many obese people. Psychosocial disadvantages reflect primarily the culture in which we find ourselves, and secondarily the people around us.

ECONOMICS

In the United States in 2009, the direct yearly medical cost of being obese was $1,723 (USD) per obese person, according to a report in *Obesity Reviews*. Being merely overweight was a relative bargain at $266. These numbers translated into $114 billion yearly, or five to 10% of total healthcare spending.

Not included in the numbers are costs such as lost productivity due to obesity-related illness and replacement or repair of items that wear out or break due to excessive amounts of physical stress. Not to mention pain and suffering.

A large majority of that money is spent on diabetes and cardiovascular disease associated with obesity. Workers who become ill due to obesity and can't go to work cost employers billions of dollars in lost productivity.

Overweight people spend at least $60 billion yearly in the United States on various weight-loss efforts.

HEALTH CONSEQUENCES

OVERALL ILLNESS AND DEATH

The numerous obesity-related illnesses are more common and severe the longer obesity has been present. And as might be expected, the fatter, the riskier. A typical high-risk person would be a 45-year-old who has weighed 260 pounds (118 kg) since the age of 20. Associated illnesses may simply cause pain (e.g., gallstones, arthritis), or contribute to premature death (e.g., heart attacks, high blood pressure).

Adverse health effects of being overweight are linked not only with total weight, but also with waist size. To measure your waist circumference, you need to know that your iliac crest is the top of the pelvis bone above your hip joint, and in most people is at about the same level as the navel. Measure your bare waist circumference at the level of the iliac crest while standing, at the end of normal breathing out, keeping the tape parallel to the floor. Women with a waist over 35 inches (89 cm), and men over 40 inches (102 cm), are at increased risk for diabetes, hypertension, high cholesterol and triglycerides, cardiovascular disease, and cancer.

Looking at all overweight and obese people as a group, the death rate is probably only mildly higher than would be expected otherwise. But the mortality rate gradually starts rising at a body mass index (BMI) of 30 (e.g., a 5-foot, 4-inch (163 cm) person weighing 174 pounds (79 kg) or a 5-foot, 10-inch (178 cm) person weighing 207 pounds or 94 kg). A major increase in medical complications and many of the premature deaths occur in those who have a body mass index over 40 (e.g., a 5-foot, 4-inch (163 cm) person weighing 240 pounds (109 kg) or a 5-foot, 10-inch (178 cm) person weighing 310 pounds or 141 kg).

You can find your own body mass index if you know your weight and height by using an online calculator such as the one at http://advancedmediterraneandiet.com/bmicalcula tor.html.

A 25-year-old morbidly obese man (e.g., 5-foot, 10-inch (178 cm) tall, 280 pounds or 127 kg)) will die 12 years sooner than otherwise expected, on average.

Obesity is involved in five of the top 10 causes of death in the United States. It's quite difficult to calculate how many U.S. deaths are directly attributable to obesity; estimates range from 112,000 to 414,000 per year.

If we look only at older Americans, over 65–75 years old, the condition of being overweight, but not obese, seems to prolong life on average. Longest life spans are seen in older Americans with a body mass index between 25 and 30. People above and below those BMIs tend to have shorter life spans.

Disability rates are lowest for older Americans with a BMI around 24. These numbers, of course, apply only to groups of people defined by BMI, not to individuals. So, if you are over 65, you may have less disability at a body mass index of 24, but you may die slightly earlier than someone with a BMI in the overweight range.

The medical complications of excessive adiposity are somewhat related to distribution of that fat on the body. The two classic distribution patterns are gynoid and android. You can have either pattern whether you are a man or a woman, although your particular pattern is hereditary.

The gynoid pattern is also referred to as lower body, femoral-gluteal, peripheral, or pear-shaped; fat is concentrated on the thighs, buttocks, hips, and lower half of the abdomen.

The android pattern is also called male-type, upper body, abdominal, central, visceral, or apple-shaped; fat is concentrated in the neck, cheeks, shoulders, and abdomen. Distribution of fat in an android or apple-shaped pattern in particular is associated with increased risk of strokes, diabetes, coronary artery disease, high blood pressure, certain cancers, and earlier death.

HIGH BLOOD PRESSURE

At least one-third of all cases of hypertension (high blood pressure) are caused by obesity. Every 20 pounds (9 kg) of excess fat causes a two to three point rise in blood pressure. If we look at people who are 20% over ideal weight, the prevalence of hypertension is twice that of normal weight people.

DIABETES MELLITUS

There are two types of diabetes mellitus. Type 1 usually starts in childhood and is fatal unless treated with insulin injections. Type 2, or adult-onset diabetes, is much more common and may be managed with diet alone, weight reduction, oral medications, and sometimes insulin. Average age at the time of diagnosis is around 50. Eighty to 90% of all type 2 diabetics are overweight.

The U.S. Centers for Disease Control and Prevention predicts that one of every three Americans born in 2000 will develop diabetes, mostly type 2.

Diabetes is easily diagnosed by finding elevated amounts of sugar (glucose) in the blood. It occurs in 11% of the adults in the United States—that's 26 million cases. In the over-65 crowd, almost one in every three has diabetes (nearly all type 2).

The high sugar levels alone can cause symptoms such as frequent urination and unusual thirst. But diabetes is clearly more complicated than simple "high sugar." Diabetes can impair circulation, nerve and kidney function, and eyesight. Although most diabetics never become blind, diabetes is a leading cause of blindness.

Risk for developing type 2 diabetes is twice the norm in those who are mildly obese, five times normal in the moderately obese, and 10 times normal in the severely obese. Duration of obesity is also an important determinant.

Having diabetes at age 50 more than doubles the risk of developing cardiovascular disease for both women and men.

Compared to those without diabetes, having both cardiovascular disease and diabetes at age 50 approximately doubles the risk of dying, regardless of sex.

Compared to those without diabetes, women and men with diabetes at age 50 die 7 or 8 years earlier, on average.

Clearly, you want to avoid diabetes if you can. One way to improve your odds is to achieve and maintain a healthy body weight.

PREDIABETES

Prediabetes is defined as 1) having fasting blood sugar between 100 and 125 mg/dl (5.56–6.94 mmol/l), or 2) having blood sugar level of 140–199 mg/dl (7.78–11.06 mmol/l) two hours after drinking 75 grams of glucose.

Overweight and obesity increase your odds of becoming prediabetic. The Centers for Disease Control in 2011 determined that 79 million Americans have prediabetes, including one in three of all adults and half of all those over 65.

Prediabetes is a strong risk factor for development of full-blown diabetes. It's also associated with increased risk for cardiovascular disease such as heart attack and stroke. One of every four adults with prediabetes develops diabetes over the next three to five years. The progression can often be prevented by lifestyle modifications such as dietary changes, moderate-intensity exercise, and modest weight loss.

GALLSTONES

Gallstones are three or four times more common in the obese. For a 5-foot, 4-inch (163 cm) tall women weighing over 174 pounds or 79 kg, the risk of developing symptomatic gallstones (belly pain, nausea, vomiting) is over 1% per year. Successful weight loss itself seems to increase the risk of symptomatic gallstones transiently.

CORONARY ARTERY DISEASE

Also known as coronary heart disease, coronary artery disease refers to complications caused by the build-up of plaque in the arteries providing the heart muscle with oxygen and nutrients. The plaque is composed of fats, cholesterol, cells, and debris. The general term for this gradual artery-blocking disease process is atherosclerosis, and it often occurs elsewhere in the body in addition to the heart.

Not uncommonly, the first sign of the problem is sudden death. More fortunate souls may just have a heart attack (aka myocardial infarction, with a 10–25% chance of dying), weakness of the heart muscle (congestive heart failure), or a heart rhythm disturbance.

In overweight people, the risk of developing coronary artery disease is directly related to the degree of fatness, starting at just 10% overweight.

The risk of heart and vascular disease is more closely associated with distribution of excess fat than with degree of obesity as measured by overall weight or body mass index. Waist-hip ratio (WHR) is a measure of abdominal or central obesity, the type of fat distribution associated with coronary artery disease. This is the android pattern discussed earlier. To determine your waist-hip ratio:

1. While standing, relax your stomach—don't pull it in. Measure around your waist midway between the bottom of the rib cage and the top of your pelvis bone. Usually this is at the level of your belly button, or an inch higher. Don't go above the rib cage. Keep the measuring tape horizontal to the ground and don't compress your skin.
2. Then measure around your hips at the widest part of your buttocks. Keep the tape horizontal to the ground and don't compress your skin.
3. Divide the waist by the hip measurement. The result is your waist-hip ratio.

For example, if your waist is 44 inches (112 cm) and hips are 48 inches (122 cm): 44 divided by 48 is 0.92, which is your waist-hip ratio.

Please take the time now to measure and note in your personal records your waist size, hip size, and calculated waist-hip ratio.

Scientists have not yet determined the ideal WHR, but it is probably around 0.85 or less for women, and 0.95 or less for men. Ratios above 1.0 are clearly associated with risk of cardiovascular disease such as heart attacks. The higher the ratio, the higher the risk. Compared with body mass index, WHR is a much stronger predictor of coronary artery disease. Several of the other obesity-related illnesses are also correlated with WHR, but the relationship between WHR and cardiovascular disease is particularly strong.

LIPIDS

Obesity tends to elevate total and LDL cholesterol, while lowering HDL cholesterol. LDL is the "bad cholesterol" and HDL is the good. These lipid changes tend to promote atherosclerosis, including coronary artery disease. Furthermore, obesity is associated with high triglycerides, which can cause painful inflammation of the pancreas and may also play a role in atherosclerosis.

CANCER

The incidence of cancer is clearly increased in people who are 40% or more over ideal weight. Men are prone to prostate and colorectal cancers. Women get cancer of the endometrium (uterus), gallbladder, cervix, ovary, and breast. Overweight and obesity are linked to increased risk of kidney cancer and esophageal adenocarcinoma. According to the American Cancer Society, overweight and obesity contribute to 14 to 20 percent of all cancer-related deaths in the United States. Over 500,000 people die from cancer each year in the United States.

RESPIRATORY PROBLEMS

In extremely overweight people, the chest wall and upper airway tissues are so thick and heavy that breathing is impaired. This results in low blood oxygen levels, brief periods during sleep in which breathing stops entirely (obstructive sleep apnea), and daytime sleepiness. My patient, Matt, from the start of this chapter, had sleep apnea.

In contrast, the shortness of breath during exertion experienced by most overweight people is just an indicator of low physical fitness or a reflection of the heavy load they haul.

MISCELLANEOUS CONSEQUENCES

A number of other medical conditions are caused by or associated with obesity:

- Strokes
- Arthritis (especially in the knees)
- Low back pain
- Gout
- Varicose veins
- Hemorrhoids
- Blood clots in the leg veins and lungs
- Complications after surgery, such as wound infection, breathing problems, blood clots, poor wound healing
- Complications during pregnancy, such as toxemia, hypertension, diabetes, prolonged labor, greater need for C-section
- Fat build-up in the liver (hepatic steatosis)
- Delayed or missed diagnosis due to difficult physical examination or weight exceeding the limit of diagnostic equipment
- Asthma
- Menstrual irregularities and decreased fertility

- Low sperm counts and testosterone levels in men

THE GOOD NEWS

Most of the medical consequences of obesity can be significantly improved by losing only 5 to 10% of your weight, sustained over time. This modest weight loss will certainly improve most cases of hypertension, diabetes, and adverse lipids. You don't have to look like a fashion model or a sexy leading man to reap the benefits of long-term weight management.

In fact, you can start very soon to take action that will eliminate or ameliorate ALL of the psychosocial, economic, and medical consequences of overweight. The process has already begun. We have just a little more groundwork to lay before getting down to nuts and bolts.

KEY POINTS

- Duration and degree of obesity are directly related to the most serious health consequences of obesity: diabetes, coronary artery disease, strokes, certain cancers, and premature death.
- Apple-shaped obese people suffer more severe medical complications than do pear-shaped.
- Most of the medical consequences of obesity can be significantly improved by losing only five to ten percent of initial body weight.

3

A Philosophy of Weight Loss

"**A**re you sure you need that dessert?" asked Amanda's husband. His not-so-subtle references to her excess weight were starting to grate on Amanda's nerves. She didn't need reminders that she was 25 to 30 pounds (11 to 14 kg) overweight. 42-year-old Amanda—5-feet, 6-inches (168 cm) tall—knew she weighed 165 pounds (75 kg).

Amanda and Jim met 13 years earlier. After a year and a half of dating, they married. It was the second marriage for both. Jim retired from the military after 20 years of service and worked as a sheriff's deputy. Amanda was an elementary teacher. She had no children of her own because of medical problems earlier in life. Jim was a good provider. He had a great sense of humor and was a God-fearing man who attended church with her. He'd send her flowers "just because." Jim liked his in-laws. He kept the yard in tip-top shape and the home in good repair. He was faithful to Amanda for the 11 years of their marriage. Not uncommonly for ex-military men, Jim could be a bit of a control freak. Amanda loved Jim anyway, and felt he loved her back. He said so. The marriage had hit a few rough patches, but the couple had worked through them successfully.

Amanda loved the outdoors. She was an avid hiker and an officer in a hiking club. Two or three weekends a month, she would take a four- to eight-mile strenuous hike either with the club or other friends. She'd strap on a 15-pound (7 kg) backpack, including camera gear for her nature photography hobby. Four days a week she'd go for a three-mile walk with her black Labrador retriever in her neighborhood. Her Lab would often tag along on her hikes carrying a first-aid kit and his own water in a dog backpack.

Amanda considered herself 15 pounds (7 kg) overweight when they married. She was 150 pounds (68 kg) at the time. Jim understood he wasn't marrying a Victoria's Secret model. She gained 10 or 15 pounds (4.5 to 7 kg) over the next five years, but had held steady since then. She's attractive, and she knows it. When she's wearing high heels and dark clothing, the extra weight disappears. Amanda eats healthy and enjoys her food. If not for Jim's comments, she'd be comfortable with her current 165 pounds (75 kg). She felt good. Several of the 20-somethings in the hiking club had trouble keeping up with her. She doesn't plan on entering the Mrs. America pageant. Everybody gains a little weight as they get older, don't they? None of her friends are at their high school weights. Few are even close.

Nevertheless, over the last couple years Jim had been increasingly critical of her weight. He could stand to lose 40 pounds (18 kg) himself. Their sex life was less active now and Amanda wasn't sure if it was related to her weight, Jim's age (47), or something else entirely. She'd catch his eyes wandering to other women more than usual. He freely shared his idea of feminine perfection with Amanda and her friends: Megan Fox. By the same token, Jim was no Brad Pitt, either. Sure, Amanda wouldn't mind being 135 pounds (61 kg) again, as thin as she was at 25. She wondered if there was an easy, painless way to get there. She wasn't excited about the sacrifices she figured were necessary to lose 30 pounds (14 kg). She'd made some half-hearted attempts at losing weight through calorie-restricted diets, without lasting success. After two or three weeks of deprivation, she couldn't stand the gnawing, unrelenting hunger. She had let Jim know many times that his derogatory weight-related comments cut her to the bone. They quarreled; he apologized. But the hurtful comments began again too soon.

Amanda and Jim's repetitive bickering about her weight started to strain their marriage. In the final analysis, she loved Jim and thought it would just be silly for her weight to jeopardize her marriage. She decided to lose 30 pounds (14 kg) and put an end to his carping. She came to see me for weight-loss pills.

THE ENERGY BALANCE EQUATION

An old joke from my medical school days asks, "How many psychiatrists does it take to change a light bulb?" Only one, but the light bulb must want to change.

How many weight-loss programs does it take before you lose that weight for good? Only one, but....

Here's the old Energy Balance Equation:

Calorie Intake minus Calories Burned
= Change in Body Fat

It's just that simple. But much easier said than done! "Calorie intake" is the food you eat or drink. "Calories burned" is the energy used in your activities and to run your body's basic life-sustaining processes (metabolism).

Your fat stores are determined by the number of calories you eat minus the calories you expend ("burn") in physical activities and resting metabolism. Obesity results from an imbalance between calorie intake and calorie expenditure. The degree of this imbalance may be quite small. Over the course of a year, all other things being equal, you'll gain three and a half pounds (1.6 kg) of fat just by adding a teaspoon (5 ml) of butter to your dinner roll every day. Simply avoid a 10-minute walk daily for a year and you'll gain five and a half pounds (2.5 kg). Taking the walk and avoiding the teaspoon of butter sound easy, but if not done you'll gain 35 pounds (16 kg) over the course of five years.

While we don't have much control over our basal metabolic energy requirements (roughly 1,200–1,500 calories daily), many of us are able to adjust food intake and activity levels to strike a happy balance in the energy equation, minimizing unwanted fat. For a lucky few, that desirable balance is automatic and unconscious. The rest of us have to think about it, work at it, make it a priority at times. I'll teach you to adjust your own energy balance equation. Right now your balance is tipped in favor of excess energy stores (fat). It will soon be tipped in the other direction. You'll convert fat to energy and lose weight in the process. Once you achieve your goal weight, the energy equation must be balanced again.

I have no doubt that the energy balance equation applies to you. People who swear they can't lose weight on extreme low-calorie diets have been locked up (with consent) in university medical center metabolic wards with access to food strictly controlled by staff. On appropriate calorie-restricted diets, everyone loses weight. When an exercise program is added, they lose more weight.

Every now and then a patient tells me he can't lose weight even though his typical daily food intake is two pieces of plain toast, a cup of grapes, a hard-boiled egg, and three celery stalks. That's 530 calories. Even if he lies around on a couch all day watching TV with a remote control channel changer, I know his basal metabolism requires at least 1,000 calories daily to keep him alive. His body must have, and will get, the extra 470 calories from his fat stores. Over time, he must lose weight as his body converts his fat into basal metabolic energy. Yet he swears he's not losing weight, and, in fact, may be gaining. I don't believe he's lying to me. What's going on here?

Researchers have clearly established that "diet resistant" dieters tend to under-estimate and under-report how much they're eating, often to a large degree. The tendency is stronger in obese folks compared to those merely overweight. The authors of my favorite study on this topic wrote that "the mechanisms responsible for this phenomenon are not well understood" (Lichtman, et al, *New England Journal of Medicine*, 1992). People who just can't lose weight despite "severe calorie restriction" are in fact eating more calories than they think.

The only way to lose weight is to cut down on the calories you take in, increase your physical activity, or do both. Although the exercise portion of the equation is somewhat optional, you must reduce food intake to lose a significant amount of weight. Once you reach your goal weight you'll be able to return to nearly your current calorie consumption, and even higher consumption if you've increased your muscle mass and continue to be active.

GRAND UNIFICATION THEORY

In the Introduction, I told you about Gary Taubes' "carbohdyrate/insulin theory of obesity." To recap: The hormone in charge of fat storage is insulin; it works to make us fatter, building fat tissue. If you've got too much fat, you must have too much insulin action. And what drives insulin secretion from your pancreas? Dietary carbohydrates, especially refined carbs such as sugars, flour, cereal grains, and starchy vegetables (e.g., corn, beans, rice, potatoes). These are the "fattening carbs." Dozens of enzymes and hormones are at play either depositing fat into tissue, or mobilizing the fat to be used as energy. It's an active process going on continuously. Any regulatory derangement that favors fat accumulation will CAUSE gluttony (overeating) or sloth (inactivity).

I think both the energy balance equation and carbohydrate/insulin theory have validity and practical application for weight management. Several studies of very-low-carbohydrate dieting show that successful dieters have reduced their calorie consumption from baseline, which supports the energy balance equation theory. By the same token, many people have lost weight on high-carbohydrate diets by reducing calories from pre-diet levels. For at least a few people, exercise does indeed accelerate the rate of weight loss. In favor of the carbohydrate/insulin theory are numerous studies finding greater degrees of weight loss, with less hunger and better compliance, on very-low-carbohydrate diets.

Undoubtedly, we all have metabolisms that differ from others because of heredity and other factors. Calorie-restricted dieting may work better for one metabolic type, whereas low-carbohydrate, eat-all-you-want dieting works better for another.

Both dieter types, however, need to incorporate willpower, commitment, knowledge, motivation, discipline, and social support. Success depends on them.

WILLPOWER AND FREE WILL

Are you able to reduce calorie intake and increase your physical activity level? Can you break your sugar-sweetened beverage habit? Will you turn down the cake and ice cream at the office party?

It boils down to whether we have free will. Free will is the power, attributed especially to humans, of making free choices that are unconstrained by external circumstances or by an agency such as divine will. Will is the mental faculty by which one chooses or decides upon a course of action; volition. Willpower is the strength of will to carry out one's decisions, wishes, or plans.

If we don't have free will, you're wasting time with this book; nothing will get your weight problem under control. Even liposuction and weight-reduction stomach surgery will fail in time if you are fated to be fat. The existence of free will is confirmed for me by my education in religion and philosophy, my intuition, and most prominently, by my experience. I suspect you wouldn't have picked up this book if you didn't believe in free will on at least some level. I have seen hundreds of my patients lose weight and keep it under control. I didn't do it for them. No other person, pill, or agency did it for them. They didn't achieve success by being passive victims of external circumstances. They cut back on calories and increased activity levels through strength of will. They did it.

COMMITMENT

Your success in weight loss and long-term management are dependent on commitment and willpower. In most cases, if not all, a change in lifestyle will be necessary. This is not easy. Your commitment and willpower will be fortified by knowledge, motivation, discipline, and social support.

KNOWLEDGE

You have learned how your body needs various nutrients, how it stores excess energy intake as fat, how it can convert fat to energy as needed for physical activity and metabolism. You know the adverse health consequences of excess fat and soon will learn about the beneficial effects of exercise. This knowledge will support your commitment and willpower.

MOTIVATION

Immediate, short-term motivation to lose weight may stem from an upcoming high school reunion, swimsuit season, or a wedding. You want to look your best. Maybe you want to attract a mate or keep one interested. Perhaps a boyfriend, co-worker, or relative said something mean about your weight. These motivators may work, but only temporarily. Basing a lifestyle change on them is like building on shifting sands. You need a firmer foundation for a lasting structure. Proper long-term motivation may grow from:

- the discovery that you feel great and have more energy when you are lighter and eating sensibly
- the sense of accomplishment from steady progress
- the acknowledgment that you have free will and are responsible for your weight and many aspects of your health
- the inspiration from seeing others take charge of their lives successfully
- the admission that you have some guilt and shame about being fat, and that you like yourself more when you're not fat
- the awareness of obesity-related health problems and their improvement with even modest weight loss.

Appropriate motivation will support your commitment and willpower.

DISCIPLINE

You already have a number of good habits that support your health and make your life more enjoyable, productive, and efficient. For example, you brush your teeth and bathe regularly, put away clean clothes in particular spots, pay bills on time, get up and go to work every day, wear your seat belt, put your keys or purse in one place when you get home, balance your checkbook periodically. At one point, these habits took much more effort than they do now. But you decided they were the right thing to do, made them a priority, practiced them at first, made a conscious effort to perform them on schedule, and repeated them over time.

All this required discipline. That's how good habits become part of your lifestyle, part of you. Over time, your habits require much less effort and hardly any thought. You just do it. Your decision to lose fat permanently means that you must establish some new habits, such as reasonable food restriction and regular exercise. You've already demonstrated that you have self-discipline. The application of that discipline to new behaviors will support your commitment and willpower.

SOCIAL SUPPORT

Success at any major endeavor is easier when you have a supportive social system. As an example, consider childhood education. A network of actors play supportive roles. Parents provide transportation, school supplies, a home study area, help with homework, etc. Siblings leave the child alone so he can do his homework, and older ones set an example. Neighbors may participate in carpooling. Taxpayers provide money for public schools. Teachers do their part. The school board oversees the curriculum, supervises teachers, and does long-range planning. Success is more likely when all the actors work together for their common goal: education of the child. Similarly, your starring role in a weight-loss program may win an Academy Award if you have a strong cast of supporting actors. Your mate, friends, co-workers, and relatives may be helpers or hindrances. It will help if they:

- give you encouragement instead of criticism
- don't tempt you with taboo food
- show respect for your commitment and will-power
- give you time to exercise
- go on a diet or exercise with you, if they're overweight or need exercise
- understand why there are no longer certain foods in the house
- appreciate the nutritious, sensible foods that are now in the house
- forgive and understand when you occasionally backslide
- gently remind you of your commitment when needed
- reward you with compliments as you make progress
- don't compare your physique unfavorably with supermodels or surgically-sculpted bodies
- don't get jealous when you lose weight and are more attractive and energetic.

Your social support system can make or break your commitment and willpower. Ask them to help you.

DIET FAILURE

Nearly everyone can lose weight on nearly any type of popular diet. Diets do work. The problem is that most people quickly regain the fat they lost. The cause usually is a breakdown of motivation, discipline, commitment, willpower, or social support, superimposed on an inadequate knowledge base.

Another type of diet failure is when the dieter gives up within the first week, even before any weight is lost.

Let me be clear: many diets deserve to fail because they're unsafe and unsustainable from a physiological viewpoint.

Let's dig further into why even reasonable diets fail so often in both the short and long run. And why are you overweight in the first place?

EVOLUTION, PHYSIOLOGY, AND OUR MODERN OBESIGENIC ENVIRONMENT

I admit it's an oversimplification to say you're fat simply because you ingested more energy (calories) than you burned up in physical activity and basal metabolism.

Why are we fat in the first place? Why do we so readily regain lost weight? For a fresh perspective, let's turn the questions around: why isn't everybody overweight? After all, throughout most of human history food has been scarce, requiring great time and physical effort to secure. During the rare times of easy food abundance, those who could locate and eat the most and store the excess as fat were better able to survive and pass their genes on to the next generation. Those who were less successful at storing energy didn't live through the next famine or were too malnourished to reproduce.

We've inherited a biological system designed to store excess energy as fat during times of abundance. The "problem" is that we now live in times of perpetual feast, not famine. Food surrounds us, marketers shower us with titillating ads, and food is cheap compared to the price "paid" by our ancestors. In our current environment, overweight is the natural condition of humankind.

PSYCHOLOGY

So why isn't everybody fat? It's because of constraints on our behavior that counteract natural tendencies. Nature tells us to eat now and eat well, for tomorrow will bring famine. So get prepared. Nature tells us to kick back and relax while we can, saving our energy for when we really need it. Like for a sprint across the savanna with a brushfire or saber-toothed tiger at our heels! For most of us who are not overweight, it is behavioral constraints that keep us from eating too much, or keep us physically active. These constraints on behavior can be divided into external and internal varieties.

External constraints are our fears of negative consequences. For example, we know or think that if we get fat there will be adverse health effects, discrimination in employment and social situations, and poorer prospects of finding and keeping a mate. Fear of these consequences keeps us exercising or from eating too much. Such fear can also be used constructively to help you lose weight and get healthier.

Internal constraints on behavior are our values or standards. To various degrees, most of us place value in achievement, productivity, discipline, knowledge, willpower, self-improvement, commitment, temperance, hygiene, and self-respect. These are the standards that shape our behaviors. When we fail to live up to the standards, guilt and shame lead us back to the right path. The potential for guilt and shame inhibits us, i.e., constrains our behavior. On a more positive note, the exhilaration of meeting the standards is its own reward, and diverts our attention from less lofty behavior. These values keep many people from overeating and get them off the couch for exercise when they'd rather watch TV. Use the values, and associated guilt and shame, to your advantage.

Most dieters on reasonable programs regain the weight they worked so hard to lose. The cause usually is a breakdown of motivation, discipline, commitment, willpower, or social support, superimposed on an inadequate knowledge base. The primary goal of this book is to boost your fund of knowledge regarding nutrition and physiology. The result will be a fortification of your motivation, discipline, commitment, and willpower. This is cognitive therapy. When faithfully applied, it works.

EMOTIONAL EATING AND PSYCHIATRIC PROBLEMS

A few overweight people have psychological problems that interfere with cognitive therapy. You may be one of them. Depression, anxiety, and other psychological disturbances can be so overwhelming as to block your ability to act on the information presented here. When you're sad, disappointed, angry, discouraged, overworked or stressed out, eating some ice cream, chocolate, cookies, or potato chips provides an immediate emotional boost and short-lived pleasure. Your subconscious remembers that boost. The next time you're upset, you eat. That's food therapy for emotional distress. But it's not the best therapy over the long haul.

Instead of reaching for food, many people find emotional relief through other avenues, such as reading, music, volunteer work, exercise, socializing, hobbies, and psychotherapy, to name a few. Careful self-examination may reveal if you're eating to satisfy emotional rather than physiological needs. If you have any doubt, or need help with emotional distress, consult a psychologist, psychiatrist, or trusted religious adviser. Awareness of the problem is half the solution.

Frequent binge eating is probably emotional. A binge is characterized by 1) eating an unusually large amount (1,500 to 20,000 calories) in an hour or two, of typically calorie-dense or "forbidden" foods, 2) a sense of lack of control over eating during the episode, and 3) feelings of disgust, depression, or guilt after overeating. The related disorder, bulimia nervosa, involves recurrent binge eating followed by inappropriate behavior to prevent weight gain, such as laxative abuse, self-induced vomiting, diuretic use, fasting, or excessive exercise. It's unclear whether binge eaters have more difficulty than anyone else during weight-loss efforts, or whether they need psychotherapy for long-term success. Habitual binge eaters generally report greater psychological distress than other obese people, and tend to have a higher incidence of personality and mood disorders such as depression.

While we're on the topic of psychology, it's important to note that successful weight loss occasionally unmasks other psychological problems. Sometimes obesity is used as a fortress to protect oneself from the outside world, allowing avoidance of intimate interaction with others. Successful weight loss can open up new social and recreational opportunities, triggering long-hidden anxieties. For instance, victims of sexual abuse may be terrified of the increasing interest shown by the opposite sex.

There are more common and less dramatic psychological drawbacks you might encounter with dieting and weight loss. Housemates may gripe unjustifiably about the food available (they shouldn't be eating that other junk anyway!). You may have to reassess your relationship with friends and co-workers who try to sabotage your diet and exercise plans. Could your spouse be a saboteur? Increased attention from the opposite sex may lead to all sorts of problems, not the least being jealousy in your spouse. Shedding pounds doesn't mean you'll shed job and relationship problems. If you thought losing 50–100 pounds (23–45 kg) would make your life magically better and problems disappear, don't let the stress of disillusionment precipitate a weight regain. Your life is better. Keep slugging away at the problem areas and you'll make progress. It's OK to ask for help.

DIET FAILURE IN TAUBES' MODEL OF OBESITY

Remember, in Taubes' model excessive carbohydrate consumption leads to excessive insulin action, which builds fat tissue. If you fail to lose weight, or regain lost weight, you're simply eating too many carbohydrates.

THE LUCKY FEW

Sure, you see people who eat all and anything they want yet don't gain weight. And they're not exercise fanatics. These lucky dogs tend to be either very physically active people, heavy smokers, or active adolescents and young adults with inherently high metabolic rates. After age 30 many of them will start developing "middle-age spread" as metabolism slows and activity levels drop. Nevertheless, it appears that one or two out of every 10 adults need not concern themselves with calories, fat grams, or counting carbohydrates—they will stay slender. Some of them have to push themselves to eat! But you and I need constraints on behavior to keep our weight under control. We're in good company. Just look around!

By the way, when the next prolonged famine hits, you'll outlive that skinny guy if you're carrying some extra fat weight.

WEIGHT GOALS

Deciding how much weight you should lose isn't as simple as it seems at first blush. I rarely have to tell a patient she's overweight. She knows it and has an intuitive sense of whether it's mild, moderate, or severe in degree. She's much less clear about how much weight she should lose. If it's any consolation, clinicians in the field aren't always sure either.

Several weight standards are in common usage:
1) Body Mass Index
2) Aesthetic Ideal Weights
3) Realistic Weights

BODY MASS INDEX

Body Mass Index (BMI) is your weight in kilograms divided by your height in meters squared (kg/m^2). A pound equals 454 kilograms. An inch equals 2.54 centimeters. There are 100 centimeters in one meter. Thus, a 5-foot, 4-inch woman (1.63 meters) weighing 200 pounds (91 kilograms) has a BMI of 34.2. Perhaps you're starting to understand why this weight standard isn't too popular yet.

To learn your own BMI but skip the math, use an online calculator such as this one:

http://advancedmediterraneandiet.com/bmicalcula
tor.html.

From a health standpoint, BMIs between 18.5 and
24.9 are the best for people under 65–75 years old.
About a third of the United States adult population
is at this healthy weight.

To see if your BMI is in the healthy range of 18.5 to
24.9, find your height in the table below, then look
to the healthy weight ranges to the right.

Table of Healthy Weight Ranges Based On Body Mass Index: 18.5 to 24.9

Height (without shoes)	Weight in lb (w/o clothes)	Weight in kg (w/o clothes)
5'0" or 152 cm	95 - 128	43.0 - 58.0
5'1" or 155 cm	98 - 132	44.4 - 59.8
5'2" or 157 cm	101 - 137	45.8 - 62.1
5'3" or 160 cm	105 - 141	47.6 - 63.9
5'4" or 163 cm	108 - 146	48.9 - 66.2
5'5" or 165 mc	111 - 150	50.3 - 68.0
5'6" or 168 cm	115 - 155	52.0 - 70.3
5'7" or 170 cm	118 - 160	53.5 - 72.5
5'8" or 173 cm	122 - 164	55.3 - 74.3
5'9" or 175 cm	125 - 169	51.7 - 76.6
5'10" or 178 cm	129 - 174	58.5 - 78.9
5'11" or 180 cm	133 - 179	60.3 - 81.8
6'0" or 183 cm	137 - 184	62.1 - 83.4
6'1" or 185 cm	140 - 189	63.5 - 85.7
6'2" or 188 cm	144 - 195	65.3 - 88.4
6'3" or 191 cm	148 - 200	67.1 - 90.7
6'4" or 193 cm	152 - 205	68.9 - 92.9

BMIs between 25 and 29.9 designate "overweight" and accurately describe about 35 percent of the United States adult population.

A BMI of 30 or higher defines "obesity" and indicates high risk for poor health. About 30 percent of us are obese. At a BMI of 35 and above, the risk of death and disease increases sharply.

The BMI concept is helpful to researchers and obesity clinicians, but the number doesn't mean much yet to the average person on the street and to many physicians. It should be used more widely. Know your BMI. If it's under 25, any excess fat you carry is unlikely to affect your health and longevity; your efforts to lose weight would be purely cosmetic.

AESTHETIC IDEAL WEIGHT

Aesthetic Ideal Weights are somewhat personal, although clearly influenced by culture. You know without much thought at what weight you look your best. Whether others agree with you, and whether you could realistically hope to reach that weight, are entirely different matters.

If your personal Aesthetic Ideal Weight matches the Hollywood hunk or sex kitten actress du jour, prepare for failure. Thespians and models want to be thin because the camera puts weight on them. Many of our beloved photogenic celebrities workout three hours daily with a personal trainer. And on top of that, many also visit plastic surgeons. I suggest you pull your head out of the stars, come back to earth, find a friend with your type of body frame and height who looks "normal" to you. What does he or she weigh? Now you've got something to shoot for. Leave the Impossible Dream to Don Quixote. I also suggest validation of your Aesthetic Ideal Weight by a trusted adviser; not someone who will say anything to boost your ego, not by an overweight girlfriend who wants to hold you back so she doesn't look bad.

REALISTIC WEIGHTS

A Realistic Weight goal is one that you have a reasonable expectation of achieving, accompanied by significant psychological or medical benefits. This standard is flexible. There is no weight chart to consult since your potential psychological or medical benefits are unique. These weights tend to be higher than the other benchmarks thus far reviewed.

Many of the illnesses caused or aggravated by obesity are improved significantly by loss of only 5 or 10% of body weight, regardless of final body mass index.

The Realistic Weight concept accepts that you can feel better, look better, and have fewer medical problems while falling far short of the healthy BMI of 18.5 to 24.9. The concept accepts that your body cannot always be shaped at will: much of your shape and fat distribution are genetically determined. For example, the transformation of a young girl into a woman is recognizable by an accumulation of fat in the right places, caused by genes beyond her control. If all your blood relatives have big buttocks, thighs, and legs, you will also, although you do have control over degree.

It's not realistic to expect a 40-year-old mother of three to look like a 17-year-old with no kids. It's clearly not impossible, but you just don't see it very often. Nor is there a need for it. The Realistic Weight concept also accounts for personal history and recognizes a point of diminishing returns, i.e., increasing effort with decreasing payoff.

For example, consider a diabetic with high blood pressure, 5-foot, 10-inches tall (178 cm), weighing 300 pounds (136 kg) for the last 20 years. His BMI is 44.5. He loses weight down to 215 pounds (98 kg), feels great, looks much better, cured his diabetes, and was able to stop one of his blood pressure medicines with his doctor's blessing. His BMI is now 31. But his body is starting to resist further weight loss. It's an increasing struggle for him, and he's not very close to his "ideal" healthy weight of 173 pounds or 79 kg (BMI 24.9). At 215 pounds (98 kg) he has gained most of the health and psychological benefits of weight loss, probably adding years to his life. 215 pounds (98 kg) isn't perfect, but it's good. He's lost 85 pounds (39 kg) of fat, which is a major accomplishment. Rejoice and be happy! For many people, the Realistic Weight concept is helpful and valid, and prevents the discouragement felt when performance falls short of ideal. Let's not allow the perfect to be the enemy of the good.

DOC, HOW MUCH WEIGHT SHOULD I LOSE?

As a medical man, I endorse the healthy BMI concept (BMI 18.5 to 24.9) while realizing you may have aesthetic reasons to shoot for the lower end of the range. If you have weight-related health issues, aim for a BMI of 18.5-24.9, with 25 to 30 as your fallback position. If you're over 65, consider a goal BMI between 25 and 30. Elderly Americans tend to live longest at BMIs of 25 to 30, although disability in that age group is lowest at a BMI of 24.

Please take the time now to measure and note in your personal records today's date and your:

Weight
Height
Waist size
Hip size
Waist-hip ratio
Current BMI
Weight goal

ARE YOU SURE YOU WANT TO LOSE WEIGHT?

The weight-loss program I recommend to you is not easy. You won't lose eight pounds (3.6 kg) of fat the first week and 20 pounds (9 kg) the first month. Progress is slow. It will require major lifestyle and attitude changes on your part, perhaps even by your household members. I realize I may scare you away and lose book sales by admitting all this, but it's the truth. Look elsewhere if you want a fast, easy solution—you'll be back. Successfully losing weight and keeping it off by any method is hard.

So why follow the Advanced Mediterranean Diet? It respects your individuality. It's relatively inexpensive. It will improve your health and sense of well-being. It's realistic and relatively convenient. It works. The program I propose to you has worked for hundreds of my patients. Sure, it's tough. But they did it. You can do it, too.

Now back to Amanda's story, from the beginning of this chapter. Her husband was hounding her to lose weight, to look more like Megan Fox. All other things being equal, she was satisfied with her weight at 165 pounds (75 kg). But his nagging and their subsequent quarreling were straining their marriage. She came to me for weight-loss pills to help her lose 30 pounds (14 kg). I found Amanda to be in perfect health, except her body mass index was mildly above the healthy range of 18.5 to 24.9. Hers was 26.7. Her strenuous hiking demonstrated the vigor of her cardiovascular, pulmonary, and musculoskeletal systems. All of her laboratory studies were normal, including cholesterol levels, triglycerides, blood sugar, and thyroid. Nearly all of her blood relatives lived to be over 85 and were robust until the end, eventually dying of "old age." I expected Amanda's health and longevity to follow the path of her relatives. I saw no medical reason for Amanda to lose weight. Any weight loss would be purely cosmetic.

I pointed out to Amanda that her net weight gain over her 11 years of marriage was only 15 pounds (7 kg), and it seemed to me Jim was blowing it all out of proportion. She had a bigger problem than 15 pounds (7 kg) of fat. I strongly suspected that the nagging and bickering were about something other than her weight. If so, losing the weight would not get to the heart of the matter, and the strain in the marriage would persist. Amanda didn't need weight-loss pills, or weight loss. I recommended they see their pastor for marital counseling. I knew the pastor had a good reputation for couples therapy, and he would be in a position to drill down to, and deal with, the core issues. Amanda and Jim needed talk therapy, not pill therapy. It turns out my hunch was correct: Jim had issues he needed to address. He did so, and the marriage improved. Among other things, the pastor recommended they spend more time together, so Jim started hiking with her regularly. He lost 20 pounds (9 kg) over the next year.

KEY POINTS

■ The only way to lose weight is to cut down on the calories you take in, increase your physical activity, or do both.

■ If you have no long-range goals and are unclear about your purpose for living, consult a spiritual adviser such as a minister, priest, or rabbi.

■ We tend to eat more and exercise less than we realize.

■ Successful weight management requires commitment, knowledge, motivation, social support, discipline, and willpower.

■ From now on, you'll have to constrain your natural eating inclinations.

■ A Realistic Weight goal is one that you have a reasonable expectation of achieving, accompanied by significant psychological or medical benefits. Oftentimes this is good enough.

■ The healthy Body Mass Index range is 18.5 to 24.9.

■ If you have medical problems caused or aggravated by obesity, aim for a Body Mass Index under 25. If that's not possible, be proud and happy with reduction to a BMI of 25 to 30, or with loss of 5 to 10% of your initial weight.

4
Two Diets: Moderate and Radical

Historically, well-respected and balanced weight-loss programs followed an established formula based on the energy balance equation. You know the drill: eat less, exercise more. This is calorie-restricted eating. Followers make moderate changes to their eating habits.

Alternatively, a radical approach to weight management is to drastically reduce consumption of fattening carbohydrates. Scientific evidence in favor of this approach has been accumulating over the last decade. This chapter explores the pros and cons of each method.

CALORIE-RESTRICTED DIETING

Reduced-calorie eating has a number of appeals. The dieter can often stick with familiar foods, which increases compliance with the program. Changes in diet can be made gradually, which appeals to many folks. A well-balanced eating plan is very safe from a health standpoint, with little risk of precipitating hair loss, lack of energy, hypoglycemia, rashes, headaches, fatigue, easy bruising, etc.

Clearly, I'm not talking about starvation diets or very-low-calorie diets here. Cutting daily calorie consumption below 1,200 for most women or below 1,500 for most men is unsustainable and possibly dangerous.

If exercise can be initiated and maintained, weight loss is enhanced. Regular physical activity while dieting can help maintain muscle mass, improve sleep patterns, improve strength and energy levels, and set the stage for a healthy lifelong exercise habit.

Calorie-restricted diets with or without an exercise component do indeed work, if followed. Sure, results may only be temporary, but that's an issue for all diets.

A major focus of mine for more than the last decade has been to educate my patients sufficiently that they'll stick with such a program and maintain their success long-term. That's a goal of this book, too. The sum total of my educational efforts is the Advanced Mediterranean Diet. It's a moderate, reduced-calorie, balanced diet with an exercise component. It's worked well for many people.

But it doesn't work for everybody. No single diet will. Advanced Mediterranean Diet non-responders and backsliders often do better with my radical Ketogenic Mediterranean Diet.

Here's a thumbnail sketch of the Advanced Mediterranean Diet. Based on your weight and sex, you're assigned a caloric intake level. Then I teach you how to approximate the traditional, healthy Mediterranean diet by eating specified amounts of whole grains, vegetables, fruits, fats, dairy products, and high-protein foods. Huge amount of variety in terms of foods and how to prepare them. I think it's a great program and have followed it myself.

However, the Advanced Mediterranean Diet is not without criticism from some quarters. One drawback is that you have to measure food and keep a fairly detailed record of consumption. If you've eaten your allocation of food for the day and you're still hungry, you can't do much about it until the next day. Weight loss tends to be slow and steady, a half to one-and-a-half pounds (0.2 to 0.7 kg) per week even though most dieters lose more in the first week. That's too slow for some folks.

That's a few of the reasons I devised the Ketogenic Mediterranean Diet. There are more.

VERY-LOW-CARBOHYDRATE DIETING

Another thumbnail sketch, this time for very-low-carb dieting. There are many different plans but they tend to share certain characteristics. If you're familiar with the Induction Phase of *Dr. Atkins New Diet Revolution*, you already know what I'm talking about.

Very-low-carb diets restrict carbohydrate consumption to 50 or fewer grams a day. This totally eliminates or drastically reduces some of our favorite foods, such as grains, beans, starchy vegetables (corn, potatoes, peas, etc), milk, and sugar. Nor can you have products made from these, such as bread, cookies, pies, cakes, potato and corn chips, and candy. You eat meat, eggs, fish, chicken, cheese, nuts, low-carb vegetables (e.g., salad greens, broccoli, green beans, cauliflower), and oils. Total calorie consumption is not restricted; you count carb grams rather than calories.

This is a radical change in eating for most people.

Numerous recent studies have demonstrated superior weight-loss results with very-low-carb diets as compared to traditional calorie-restricted diets. Weight loss is often faster and more consistently in the range of one or two pounds (0.5 to 0.9 kg) a week. Very-low-carb dieters have less trouble with hunger. If you do get hungry, there's always something you can eat. From a practical, day-to-day viewpoint, these diets can be easier to follow, with a bit less regimentation than calorie-restricted plans.

Sounds great! So why aren't very-low-carb diets used more often? Many dieters can't live with the restrictions. Your body may rebel against the switch from a carbohydrate-based energy metabolism to one based on fats. Most of us live in a society or sub-culture in which carbohydrates are everywhere and they're cheap; temptation is never-ending.

Just as calorie-restricted diets aren't for everybody, neither are very-low-carb diets. Some people respond to one or the other of the diet styles, others do well with either. With dieting, a one-size-fits-all approach is not the best. If it's safe, why not give folks a choice?

I've been an advocate of the traditional Mediterranean diet for the general public for over a decade. By "diet" in this context, I mean a person's usual way of eating, not a weight-loss program. In 2009, I took a close look at the individual components of the traditional Mediterranean diet and noted that many of them could be incorporated into a very-low-carbohydrate weight-loss diet. My idea was to combine the health benefits of the Mediterranean diet with the potential weight-loss benefits of very-low-carb diets. The result is the Ketogenic Mediterranean Diet.

ADVANCED OR KETOGENIC MEDITERRANEAN: HOW DO I CHOOSE?

Perhaps you have a strong preference already, just based on the thumbnail sketches. Don't ignore your intuition, but consider some other factors. Remember, you're not making an irrevocable life-long decision. If your first choice doesn't suit you, try the other. Both plans work if you follow them. Some of my patients flip back and forth from one to the other, depending on their goals.

CHOOSE THE ADVANCED MEDITERRANEAN DIET IF . . .

- you want to capture the proven maximal health benefits of the Mediterranean diet
- you're a conservative, traditional type of person
- slower weight loss is acceptable
- you have any doubts about your underlying healthiness and strength

- you still believe that dietary total fat, saturated fat, and cholesterol promote heart and vascular disease
- you have gout, chronic kidney disease, or major chronic liver disease
- you just know you can't restrict carbohydrates drastically
- you've already tried and failed very-low-carb diets
- you don't like fish
- you enjoy the ultimate in variety

CHOOSE THE KETOGENIC MEDITERRANEN DIET IF . . .

- the potential for faster and easier weight loss appeals to you
- you're certain you're completely healthy and vigorous
- you think you can live with major carbohydrate restriction
- you've done well with very-low-carb eating in the past
- you prefer less regimentation
- you've suffered much hunger on calorie-restricted diets in the past
- you're not going to exercise
- you love salads and vinaigrettes
- you enjoy a glass of wine
- you don't have gout, chronic kidney disease, or major chronic liver disease

My gut feeling is that eating closer to the traditional Mediterranean diet, as opposed to very-low-carb eating, is probably the healthier way to go long-term. But we don't really know for sure. The two styles have never been compared head-to-head in a well-designed, multi-year, scientific study to answer the question: which is healthier?

5

The Ketogenic Mediterranean Diet

INTRODUCTION

If you chose the Advanced Mediterranean Diet, shoot on over to chapter seven and skip chapters five (this one) and six.

I originally devised the very-low-carbohydrate Ketogenic Mediterranean Diet specifically for my patients with one or more of the following conditions:

- type 2 diabetes
- prediabetes
- metabolic syndrome

As it turns out, the Ketogenic Mediterranean Diet also works quite well for otherwise healthy people who are just overweight or obese.

Diabetes and prediabetes always involve impaired carbohydrate metabolism: ingested carbs are not handled by the body in a healthy fashion, leading to high blood sugars and, eventually, poisonous complications.

"Metabolic syndrome" may be a new term for you. It's a constellation of clinical factors that are associated with increased future risk of type 2 diabetes and atherosclerotic complications such as heart attack and stroke. One in six Americans has metabolic syndrome. Diagnosis requires at least three of the following five conditions:

1. high blood pressure (130/85 or higher, or using a high blood pressure medication)
2. low HDL cholesterol: under 40 mg/dl (1.03 mmol/l) in a man, under 50 mg/dl (1.28 mmol/l) in a women (or either sex taking a cholesterol-lowering drug)
3. triglycerides over 150 mg/dl (1.70 mmol/l) (or taking a cholesterol-lowering drug)
4. abdominal fat: waist circumference 40 inches (102 cm) or greater in a man, 35 inches (89 cm) or greater in a woman
5. fasting blood glucose over 100 mg/dl (5.55 mmol/l)

Metabolic syndrome and simple excess weight often involve impaired carbohydrate metabolism. Over time, excessive carbohydrate consumption can turn overweight and metabolic syndrome into prediabetes, then type 2 diabetes.

In their 2011 book, *The Art and Science of Low Carbohydrate Living*, Drs. Jeff Volek and Stephen Phinney blame our epidemic of overweight on "carbohydrate intolerance." That's a more succinct way of saying "impaired carbohydrate metabolism," a phrase I used above to characterize diabetes, pre-diabetes, and many cases of metabolic syndrome. You may recall from an earlier chapter Gary Taubes' answer as to why we get fat: excessive carbohydrate consumption, leading to high insulin release by the pancreas, leading to build-up of fat tissue. In other words, the carbohydrate/insulin theory of obesity.

The key feature of the Ketogenic Mediterranean Diet is carbohydrate restriction, which directly addresses impaired carbohydrate metabolism naturally.

My primary goal with this program—the world's first very-low-carb Mediterranean diet—is to reap the health benefits of Mediterranean-style eating while losing excess fat weight.

Secondary goals, which may not apply to you, are control of blood sugars in diabetics and prediabetics, and cure of metabolic syndrome.

The Ketogenic Mediterranean Diet usually works very well in controlling blood sugar levels in people with diabetes. So well, in fact, that diabetics taking drugs to control blood sugars may need to reduce drug dosages drastically. This should only be done under the supervision of a personal physician familiar with all medical details of the diabetic. You can find details about use of the Ketogenic Mediterranean Diet for diabetics at http://DiabeticMediterraneanDiet.com, or in my 2011 book, *Conquer Diabetes and Prediabetes: The Low-Carb Mediterranean Diet.*

WHY "KETOGENIC"?

Your body gets nearly all its energy either from fats, or from carbohydrates like glucose and glycogen. In people eating normally, 60% of their energy at rest comes from fats. In a ketogenic diet, the carbohydrate content of the diet is so low that the body has to break down even more of its fat to supply energy needed by most tissues. Fat breakdown generates ketone bodies in the bloodstream. Hence, "ketogenic diet." Also called "very-low-carb diets," ketogenic diets have been around for over a hundred years.

Ketogenic diets have several practical advantages over other diets (disputed by some authorities):
- simplicity
- almost unlimited access to many high-protein and fatty foods
- less trouble with hunger
- better short-term weight loss than many other diets (long-term, too?)
- lower blood sugar levels, which is important to people with diabetes, prediabetes, and metabolic syndrome
- reduced insulin levels in people who often have elevated levels (hyperinsulinemia), which may help reduce chronic diseases like type 2 diabetes, high blood pressure, some cancers, and coronary heart disease
- higher levels of HDL cholesterol and lower triglycerides, which may reduce risk of heart disease
- it obviously works well for a significant portion of the overweight population, but not for everybody
- better adherence to the program compared with other diets, at least for the short-term

WHY "MEDITERRANEAN"?

For years, the Mediterranean diet has been widely recognized as the healthiest diet for the general population. The enduring popularity of the Mediterranean diet is attributable to three things:

1. Taste
2. Variety
3. Health benefits

(In this context, I'm using "diet" to refer to the usual food and drink of a person, not a weight-loss program.)

The scientist most responsible for the popularity of the diet, Ancel Keys, thought the heart-healthy aspects of the diet were related to low saturated fat consumption. He also thought the lower blood cholesterol levels in Mediterranean populations (at least Italy and Greece) had something to do with it, too. Dietary saturated fat does tend to raise cholesterol levels.

Even if Keys was wrong (and I think he was) about saturated fat and cholesterol levels being positively associated with heart disease, numerous studies indicate that the Mediterranean diet is one of the healthiest around. The research involved eight countries on three continents, so it's not just a Mediterranean climate or geography effect.

Strong evidence supports the Mediterranean diet's association with:

- increased lifespan
- lower rates of cardiovascular disease such as heart attacks and strokes
- lower rates of cancer (prostate, breast, uterus, colon)
- lower rates of dementia
- lower incidence of type 2 diabetes

Weaker supporting evidence links the Mediterranean diet with:

- slowed progression of dementia
- prevention of melanoma (serious skin cancer)
- lower severity of type 2 diabetes, as judged by diabetic drug usage and blood sugar levels
- less risk of developing obesity
- better blood pressure control in the elderly
- improved weight loss and weight control in type 2 diabetics
- improved control of asthma
- reduced risk of developing diabetes after heart attack
- reduced risk of mild cognitive impairment
- prolonged life of Alzheimer disease patients
- lower rates and severity of chronic obstructive pulmonary disease lower risk of gastric (stomach) cancer
- less risk of macular degeneration in the eye
- less Parkinsons disease
- increased chance of pregnancy in women undergoing fertility treatment
- reduced prevalence of metabolic syndrome (when supplemented with nuts)
- lower incidence of asthma and allergy-like symptoms in children of women who followed the Mediterranean diet while pregnant

So what exactly is this traditional, healthy "Mediterranean diet"? Here are the predominant features:
- it maximizes natural whole foods and minimizes highly processed ones
- small amounts of red meat
- less than four eggs per week
- low to moderate amounts of poultry and fish
- daily fresh fruit
- seasonal locally grown foods with minimal processing

- concentrated sugars only a few times per week
- wine in low to moderate amounts, and usually taken at mealtimes
- milk products (mainly cheese and yogurt) in low to moderate amounts
- olive oil as the predominant fat
- abundance of foods from plants: vegetables, fruits, beans, potatoes, nuts, seeds, breads and other whole grain products
- naturally low in saturated fat, trans fats, and cholesterol
- naturally high in fiber, phytonutrients, vitamins (e.g., folate), antioxidants, and minerals (especially when compared with concentrated, refined starches and sugars in a modern Western diet)
- naturally high in monounsaturated and polyunsaturated fats, particularly as a replacement for saturated fats

WHAT'S WRONG WITH PURE MEDITERRANEAN?

The traditional Mediterranean diet derives most of its calories from carbohydrates—anywhere from 45 to 60% of total energy. If the carbohydrate/insulin theory of obesity is correct, all those carbs could lead to excessive insulin release, leading in turn to storage of calories as fat tissue. For those trying to lose weight, the insulin could impair our ability to turn that fat into weightless energy.

The Ketogenic Mediterranean Diet removes most of the carbohydrates in the traditional Mediterranean diet, lowering insulin levels, allowing fat tissue to break down and supply us with energy. The very-low-carb Ketogenic Mediterranean Diet is also compatible with Volek and Phinney's "carbohydrate intolerance" model of overweight.

Despite an emphasis on carb-rich bread, pasta, fruits, legumes, and certain vegetables, the traditional Mediterranean diet has several healthy components compatible with a very-low-carb eating style:

- olive oil
- nuts and seeds
- low-carbohydrate vegetables
- low-carbohydrate fruits
- eggs
- chicken
- meat
- wine
- fish
- cheese
- Mediterranean spices

POTENTIAL PROBLEMS WITH VERY-LOW-CARB EATING

Long-term effects of a very-low-carb or ketogenic diet in most people are unclear. They may have better or worse overall health; we just don't know for sure yet. Perhaps some people gain a clear benefit, while others—with different metabolisms and genetic make-up—are worse off.

If the diet results in major weight loss that lasts, we may see longer lifespan, less type 2 diabetes, less cancer, less heart disease, less high blood pressure, and fewer of the other obesity-related medical conditions.

Ketogenic diets are generally higher in protein, total fat, saturated fat, and cholesterol than some other diets, at least in terms of percentages. Some authorities are concerned this may increase the risk of coronary heart disease and stroke; the latest evidence indicates otherwise (see Selected References at the back of the book).

Some authorities worry that ketogenic diets have the potential to cause kidney stones, osteoporosis (thin, brittle bones), gout, deficiency of vitamins and minerals, and may worsen existing kidney disease. Others disagree.

It's clear that compliance with very-low-carb diets is difficult to maintain for six to 12 months. In other words, it's hard to stick with it. Many folks can't do it for more than a couple weeks. Potential long-term effects, therefore, haven't come into play for most users. When used for weight loss, regain of lost weight is a problem, but regain is a major issue with all weight-loss programs. I anticipate that the majority of non-diabetics who try a ketogenic diet will stay on it for only one to six months. After that, more carbohydrates can be added to gain the potential long-term benefits of additional fruits and vegetables, legumes, and whole grains. Or not.

People with type 2 diabetes or prediabetes may be so pleased with the metabolic effects of the ketogenic diet that they'll stay on it long-term.

MORE ON CARBOHYDRATE INTOLERANCE

Diabetics, prediabetics, and many folks with metabolic syndrome must remember that their bodies do not, and cannot, handle dietary carbs in a normal, healthy fashion. In a way, carbs are toxic to them. Toxicity may lead to amputations, blindness, kidney failure, nerve damage, poor circulation, frequent infections, premature heart attacks and death, among other things.

Diabetics and prediabetics simply don't tolerate carbs in the diet like other people. If you don't tolerate something, you have to give it up, or at least cut way back on it. Lactose-intolerant individuals give up milk and other lactose sources. Celiac disease patients don't tolerate gluten, so they give up wheat and other sources of gluten. One of every five high blood pressure patients can't handle normal levels of salt in the diet; they have to cut back or their blood pressure's too high. Patients with phenylketonuria don't tolerate phenylalanine and have to restrict foods that contain it. If you're allergic to penicillin, you have to give it up. If you don't tolerate carbs, you have to give them up or cut way back. I'm sorry.

PRECAUTIONS AND DISCLAIMER

The ideas and suggestions in this book are provided as general educational information only and should not be construed as medical advice or care. Information herein is meant to complement, not replace, any advice or information from your personal health professional. All matters regarding your health require supervision by a personal physician or other appropriate health professional familiar with your current health status. Always consult your personal physician before making any dietary or exercise changes. Steve Parker, M.D., and the publisher disclaim any liability or warranties of any kind arising directly or indirectly from use of this diet. If any medical problems develop, always consult your personal physician. Only your physician can provide you medical advice. You should not follow this diet if you are a child, pregnant or lactating, have alcoholism or history of alcohol abuse, have abnormal liver or kidney function, or have gout or a high uric acid blood level. Your physician may have to adjust medication dosages—particularly blood pressure pills and diabetic drugs—if you follow this diet.

LET'S GET STARTED!

The Ketogenic Mediterranean Diet is a very-low-carb diet—20 to 40 grams of digestible carbohydrate daily—designed for loss of excess body fat and control of high blood sugars. "Digestible carbohydrate" is the total carbohydrate grams minus the fiber grams of carbohydrate that you can't digest and utilize as an energy source.

For you nutrition science geeks, here's the macronutrient breakdown. Of the total calories eaten, 7–10% are from carbohydrate, 55–65% are from fat, 22–30% are from protein, and 5–10% are from alcohol.

You'll find a three-page printable version of the basic Ketogenic Mediterranean Diet (KMD) here: http://advancedmediterraneandiet.com/printabledo cuments.html.

HERE'S WHAT YOU'LL EAT:

1) Unlimited fish, meat, chicken, turkey, eggs, shrimp, lobster
2) Fish, at least 4 oz (115 g) daily
3) Olive oil, virgin or extra-virgin, at least 2–3 tbsp (30–45 ml) daily
4) Nuts and seeds, 1 oz (28 g) daily
5) Vegetables, up to 14 oz (400 g) daily
6) Wine, 6–12 fl oz (180–360 ml) daily (see alternatives in Miscellaneous Comments)
7) Cheese, up to 3 oz (85 g) daily, optional
8) Daily supplements:
   - 1 or 2 plain Centrum multivita-

min/multimineral supplements (two if over 250 lb or 114 kg)
- Magnesium oxide 250 mg
- Calcium carbonate 500 mg elemental calcium (500 mg twice daily if over 250 lb or 114 kg)
- Extra vitamin D to reach total of 1,000–1,200 IU (each Centrum has 400 IU)
- Potassium gluconate 2,750 mg (450 mg elemental potassium) or Morton Salt Substitute (potassium chloride) ¼ tsp (1.2 g)
- If prone to constipation: sugar-free Metamucil powder 1–2 rounded tsp (5.8–11.6 g) in water
- At least three quarts or liters of water

What makes it Mediterranean? Natural whole foods, fish, olive oil, nuts, wine, cheese, spices.

What's not Mediterranean? Unlimited meat and animal proteins, and absence of most sweet fruits, high-carbohydrate vegetables, potatoes, grains, legumes, pasta, honey, and yogurt. These may come later.

You can track your blood sugars and consumption of the major foods with the "KMD & LCMD Daily Log" available free at http://advancedmediterraneandiet.com/printabledo cuments.html

See chapter eight for "A Week of Meals" consistent with the Ketogenic Mediterranean Diet. Or just use your imagination while following the guidelines above.

WARNING

Wine and other alcoholic beverages are dangerous. You should not drink wine or any alcohol if you have a history of alcohol abuse or alcoholism, have liver or pancreas disease, are pregnant or trying to become pregnant, may have the need to operate dangerous equipment or machinery—such as driving a car—while under the influence of alcohol, or have demonstrated inability to limit yourself to acceptable intake levels.

FOOD CATEGORY COMMENTS:

1. Protein Group

This includes fish, meat, chicken, turkey, eggs, shrimp, lobster, and fried pork skins. Try to avoid overly processed protein products; aim for pure and simple. Processed meats may have added carbohydrates, nitrites, and other chemicals you don't need. Canned products are OK. *Eat until full or satisfied, not stuffed.*

2. Fish

Canned fish may be more affordable and convenient. Cold-water fatty fish have more of the healthy omega-3 fatty acids: trout, salmon, sardines, mackerel, albacore/white tuna, herring, swordfish, halibut, and sea bass. If you're pregnant, trying to become pregnant, or a nursing mother, avoid eating king mackerel, swordfish, shark, and tilefish (sold as golden snapper or golden bass); these fish may contain amounts of mercury harmful to breast-fed infants and babies in the womb. If you eat lots of locally caught freshwater fish, especially if you are a woman of childbearing age, check with your regional governmental authorities regarding contaminants. In the U.S., the appropriate state agency is usually the Health Department or Game and Fish Department. Note that adult medical problems attributable to chemical fish contamination are exceedingly rare in the U.S.

3. Olive oil

Use virgin or extra virgin oil in vinaigrette or other olive oil-based salad dressing. Sauté with it. Fry eggs and steak with it. Drink it straight if you want!

4. Nuts and Seeds

Almonds, walnuts, pecans, Brazil nuts, hazelnuts (filberts), macadamia nuts, peanuts (a legume), Spanish peanuts, pistachios, pine nuts, sunflower seeds, pumpkin seeds in shells. These average 3 g of digestible carbohydrate per ounce (28 g). Sunflower seeds, peanuts, and pistachios are the highest-carb: 3.5 to 4 g per ounce (28 g). Sorry, no cashews.

5. Vegetables & Fruit

(A) Raw salad vegetables: lettuce, mushrooms, radishes, spinach, alfalfa sprouts, cucumber, tomato, scallions, parsley, jicama, arugula, endive, radicchio, chard, sweet peppers, avocado, olives (pickled green or ripe black), pickles (dill or sour, not sweet or "bread and butter"). Average digestible carbohydrate per 7 oz serving (200 g) is 5 g. The highest digestible carb counts are in scallions and jicama (8 g), and sweet peppers (7g).

(B) Solid vegetables, often cooked: snow peas, broccoli, summer squash, tomato, onion, cauliflower, eggplant, Brussels sprouts, asparagus, okra, sauerkraut (canned), green beans. These average 8 g of digestible carbohydrate per 7 oz serving (200 g). Onion is highest at 14 g. Weigh these before cooking.

6. Wine

Red wine (e.g., Burgundy, Cabernet Sauvignon, or Merlot) may be healthier than white (e.g., Sauvignon Blanc, Riesling, Pinot Grigio). One fl oz (30 ml) of wine has 1 g of carbohydrate.

7. Cheese

Real, regular cheese; not low-fat. Mozzarella, provolone, Swiss, cheddar, blue, Monterey, Colby, Brie, Parmesan, feta, Gouda, ricotta, cottage. These have 1 g carbohydrate per oz (28 g). Other cheeses have too many carbs.

MISCELLANEOUS COMMENTS:

Alternatives to wine (choose only one daily):
- Extra 200 g (7 oz) vegetables, and consider a grape extract supplement daily, or
- 20 g (0.7 oz) of dark chocolate (65-85% cacao) daily, or
- Beer, 12 fl oz (360 ml) daily, but must have under 10 g of carbs, or
- Distilled spirits (whiskey, rum, vodka, gin), 80 proof, 1.5 fl oz (45 ml) daily

Additional daily optional oils, spices, and condiments (unlimited unless noted):

Butter, plant oils (strongly favor olive oil), vinegar (cider, red wine, or distilled), balsamic vinegar (2 tsp or 10 ml daily), salt, pepper, genuine mayonnaise (not low-fat), yellow mustard (1 tbsp or 15 ml daily), salad dressing (with three or fewer grams of carbohydrate per 2 tbsp or 30 ml) (2 tbsp daily), Worcestershire sauce (1 tbsp or 15 ml), A.1. Steak Sauce (1 tbsp or 15 ml)

Prominent Mediterranean spices: paprika, cumin, turmeric, cinnamon, ginger (0.35 oz or 10 g raw root, or 2 tsp or 10 ml ground spice daily), coriander, anise, Spanish saffron, lemon or lime juice (2 tbsp or 30 ml daily), mint, parsley, garlic (3 cloves daily), dill pepper, and sumac

Tea and coffee in moderation are fine. Don't add milk to them; use full-fat cream or high-fat half-and-half.

All of the recommended supplements are readily available at supermarkets and pharmacies at a reasonable cost.

I recommend Centrum for people on the Ketogenic Mediterranean Diet. Why Centrum? It's been around for years and has a good reputation. It's widely available at a reasonable price. A different brand of multivitamin/multimineral supplement may be fine if it's close to Centrum's components. Since the composition of plain Centrum could change at any time (or be concocted differently in non-U.S. countries), listed below are the contents of the U.S. product in 2011. Here are the component amounts with "% Daily Values" in parentheses:

Vitamin A 3,5000 IU (70%), Vitamin C 60 mg (100%), Vitamin D 400 IU (100%), Vitamin E 30 IU (100%), Vitamin K 25 mcg (31%), Thiamin 1.5 mg (100%), Riboflavin 1.7 mg (100%), Niacin 20 mg (100%), Vitamin B6 2 mg (100%), Folic Acid 400 mcg (100%), Vitamin B12 6 mcg (100%), Biotin 30 mcg (10%), Pantothenic Acid 10 mg (100%), Calcium 200 mg (20%), Iron 18 mg (100%), Phosphorus

20 mg (2%), Iodine 150 mcg (100%), Magnesium 50 mg (13%), Zinc 11 mg (73%), Selenium 55 mcg (79%), Copper 0.5 mg (25%), Manganese 2.3 mg (115%), Chromium 35 mcg (29%), Molybdenum 45 mcg (60%), Chloride 72 mg (2%), Potassium 80 mg (2%), Boron 75 mcg, Nickel 5 mcg, Silicon 2 mg, Tin 10 mcg, Vanadium 10 mcg.

U.S. government authorities recommend Percent Daily Values for average non-pregnant healthy adults eating 2,000 calorie a day.

Need a sweet, crunchy treat? Metamucil Fiber Wafers (12 g each), two per week.

Don't just eat the same eight or 10 items—aim for great variety. For meal ideas, see chapter seven for a week of meals and special recipes.

You'll be eating lots of salad.

You'll need a scale to measure your vegetables and to follow the optional recipes in chapter seven.

To make your food shopping easier, you can print a grocery shopping list of all foods on the Ketogenic and Low-Carb Mediterranean Diets when you visit this web page: http://advancedmediterraneandiet.com/printabledo cuments.html

WHAT COULD GO WRONG?

Very-low-carb ketogenic diets have been associated with headaches, bad breath, easy bruising, nausea, fatigue, aching, muscle cramps, constipation, and dizziness, among other symptoms. "Induction flu" may occur around days two through five, consisting of achiness, easy fatigue, and low energy. It usually clears up after a few days.

Very-low-carb ketogenic diets may have the potential to cause osteoporosis (thin, brittle bones), kidney stones, low blood pressure, constipation, gout, high uric acid in the blood, excessive loss of sodium and potassium in the urine, worsening of kidney disease, deficiency of calcium and vitamins A, B, C, and D, among other adverse effects.

Athletic individuals who perform vigorous exercise should expect a deterioration in performance levels during the first three to four weeks of any ketogenic very-low-carb diet. The body needs that time to adjust to burning mostly fat for fuel rather than carbohydrate.

Competitive weight-lifters or other anaerobic athletes (e.g., sprinters) may be hampered by the low muscle glycogen stores that accompany ketogenic diets. They may need more carbohydrates.

WHAT'S NEXT?

I recommend that anyone trying the Ketogenic Mediterranean Diet give it at least an eight to twelve week trial. Then evaluate whether it's time to move on to higher carbohydrate consumption. Remember, the KMD provides 20 to 40 grams of carbohydrate daily. Everyone has a different level of "carbohydrate intolerance" that leads to fat weight gain. It takes experimentation to find your personal intolerance level. Many people find that if they exceed 80 to 100 grams daily, they gain back the lost weight. See chapter 11 for advice on transitioning to higher carbohydrate consumption and long-term maintenance of weight loss.

6
Daily Life With Low-Carb Eating

I haven't scared you off yet, huh?

Great!

If you've chosen to follow the Advanced rather than Ketogenic Mediterranean diet, this chapter is not for you; go to chapter seven. KMD followers, read on.

The very-low-carbohydrate program I've laid out presents some definite challenges, a few of which are unique. Think of them as opportunities for personal growth. But you don't have to go it alone, nor blaze any trails through uncharted territory. I'm here to help, as is a scattered online low-carb community.

This chapter will give you an approach to overcoming the common problems linked to low-carb eating. The coping mechanisms here are not exhaustive, and you'll need, at times, to figure out for yourself what works for you and your unique metabolism.

In order, here's what's ahead:

1. Find more low-carb recipes
2. Short-term physical effects
3. Shopping for food
4. Dining out
5. Cheating
6. Sweet cravings
7. Holidays
8. Hunger
9. Record-keeping
10. Weight-loss tips
11. Social issues

1. FIND MORE LOW-CARB RECIPES

Chapter eight has a few low-carb recipes, in the "A Week of Meals" and "Special Recipes" sections. Find many more at free low-carb websites and online forums, such as:

- The message boards at Low Carb Friends (http://www.lowcarbfriends.com)
- Active Low-Carbers Forum (http://forum.lowcarber.org)
- Laura Dolson's About.com: Low Carb Diets blog (http://lowcarbdiets.about.com)
- Chef Barrae has posted hundreds of low-carb recipes (including nutritional analysis) at her blog: Unrestricted Tastes on Restricted Diets: Distinctive Diabetic Recipes (http://chefbarrae.blogspot.com).

- Jennifer Eloff has authored numerous low-carb cookbooks, starting with her flagship, *Splendid Low-Carbing*, followed by four others in the same vein. Jennifer generously shares many of her fantastic recipes at her blog, Splendid Low-Carbing. Most of her recipes include some nutrient analysis, such as carb and calorie counts. Jennifer has a particular interest in cooking with Splenda, helping you satisfy your sweet tooth. Find her blog at (http://low-carb-news.blogspot.com/).

- DAR, a type 2 diabetic, offers her favorite low-carb recipes at http://dardreams.wordpress.com/. Nutrient analysis is limited to digestible carb grams, referred to as "net carbs."

- Dana Carpender has a number of great low-carb recipe books, such as the classic *500 Low-Carb Recipes*, as well as *200 Low-Carb Slow Cooker Recipes*, *15-Minute Low-Carb Recipes*, and *1001 Low-Carb Recipes*. Check out some of her free online recipes and purchase books at her blog, Hold the Toast! (http://holdthetoast.com/).

- All Day I Dream About Food (http://dreamaboutfood.blogspot.com/). Carolyn Ketchum, a blogger with prediabetes, shares her low-carb and/or gluten-free recipes.

Among the numerous low-carb cookbooks available, a great place to start is *Low-Carbing Among Friends*, volume 1, by Jennifer Eloff, Maria Emmerich, Carolyn Ketchum, Lisa Marshall, and Kent Altena. All 325 recipes are gluten-free and low-carb (10 or fewer grams per serving).

You need to know the digestible or *net carb grams* per serving of any recipe you try. If not provided for you, you can do a full nutritional analysis of any recipe at SELF-NutritionData (http://nutritiondata.self.com/).

2. SHORT-TERM PHYSICAL EFFECTS

Very-low-carb eating is quite safe in the vast majority of generally healthy people. However, you need to be aware of minor problems that may crop up.

INDUCTION FLU

This refers to a sense of mild malaise, easy-fatigue, low energy, achiness, and dizziness that often affects people switching from a carbohydrate-based energy metabolism to fat-based. Some folks have the entire syndrome, others just parts. It starts on the second or third day of the diet and may last for several days, a week at the most. People with diabetes need to make sure the symptoms are not caused by low blood sugar by using their home glucose monitor.

Regarding low energy and easy fatigue, people who are used to exercising or working vigorously may notice that they can't perform at their prior workload, an effect that may be noticeable for two to four weeks. They may need to cut back the intensity of their work-outs temporarily. The first few weeks of very-low-carb eating are not a good time to start a vigorous exercise program.

Induction flu is temporary. It's proof that your body is going through a watershed moment. Try to tough it out—you'll be glad you did.

LEG CRAMPS

These occur commonly in the first few weeks or months. They tend to happen at night, even waking people from sleep. While not serious, they can be painful. Cramps are often prevented by taking additional supplemental magnesium, potassium, calcium, or a combination. If they persist, see your doctor for a blood test of these minerals.

A stretching exercise may prevent leg cramps: 1) Stand about two or three feet away from a wall (measured at the toes) and keep your feet planted in one spot, 2) lean forward against the wall and use your outstretched arms and hands to keep your body from hitting the wall, 3) keeping your trunk and legs in a straight line, bend your elbows to let your head approach the wall, 4) notice the slight tensing and stretching of the calf muscles (this may be slightly uncomfortable but shouldn't be painful), 5) hold that position for 10 seconds, 6) then stand up straight and relax a while, 7) repeat steps 1 through 5 for five or ten times. For nocturnal leg cramps, do this stretching just before bedtime.

CONSTIPATION OR DIARRHEA

If a bowel problem occurs, it's more likely to be constipation related to lower-than-usual fiber consumption. Others have the opposite problem, diarrhea. You might be able to identify a specific food causing symptoms, such as cheese and constipation. Eliminate or cut back on the offending item. Sugar-free Metamucil powder—one teaspoon in water—once or twice daily usually resolves constipation. Or you could concentrate on the higher fiber vegetables.

LOW BLOOD SUGAR

Since ingested carbohydrates are normally the main source of blood sugar, cutting back drastically tends to reduce blood sugar levels, even in people who don't have diabetes or prediabetes. Symptoms of low blood sugar (hypoglycemia) are rare in healthy people starting a ketogenic diet. But hypoglycemia is much more common and potentially serious in diabetics taking certain medications.

LOW BLOOD PRESSURE

The Ketogenic Mediterranean Diet is relatively low in salt, which may explain why low blood pressure can occur. If you take drugs to lower your blood pressure, the dosage my need to be reduced to prevent excessively low blood pressure. Symptoms of low blood pressure include dizziness, lightheadedness, weakness, fainting, and fatigue. Note the similarity to induction flu. You may notice these only when going from sitting to standing, or from lying to standing.

If low blood pressure is causing the symptom, we usually find a systolic blood pressure under 90 mmHg. "Systolic pressure" is the top or first number in a blood pressure reading such as 125/85 (systolic pressure is 125). The only way to tell if the aforementioned symptoms are related to blood pressure is to check a blood pressure with an accurate monitor, which most of us don't have at home or work. Perhaps you could borrow a friend's. Alternatively, check your blood pressure at your doctor's office or one of the free machines in many pharmacies and supermarkets. In those settings, a systolic pressure under 100 mmHg, even if you feel fine, suggests that your pressure at other times is under 90. Low blood pressures often responds to an increase in salt and water consumption, such as half a teaspoon daily mixed in water or used on food.

3. SHOPPING

Finding food for the Ketogenic Mediterranean Diet shouldn't be a problem. Specific recommended foods are readily available at supermarkets. People committed long-term to the low-carb way of eating often get into baking or cooking with low-carb components that may be a bit harder to find. An example is almond flour, used as a substitute for wheat flour in baking cookies and pastries, among other things. You may find low-carb products at local stores or available on the Internet (e.g., Netrition.com).

You'll find a grocery shopping list for the Ketogenic and Low-Carb Mediterranean Diets at this URL: http://advancedmediterraneandiet.com/printabledo cuments.html.

How to choose a fresh fish for cooking:

1. Sniff it. Pass if it smells fishy, nasty, or pungent.
2. Check for clear, dark eyes. Pass if eyes are dull gray and sunken.
3. Does it look or feel slimy? Take a pass.
4. Skin should be moist and shiny, almost metallic.
5. Flesh should be firm, not mushy. Press it with your finger—it shouldn't leave an imprint.
6. Look for bright red gills.
7. Cook within a day or two.

Keep your refrigerator and cupboards stocked with the foods you'll be eating, particularly if others in your household are eating regular high-carb foods that will tempt you.

4. DINING OUT

You'll be tempted to return to "normal" high-carb eating especially when you're away from your home's well-stocked cupboards and refrigerator. Be ready to deal with it.

One option is to take your food with you. For road trips, take nuts, dark chocolate, canned fish and meat, vegetables, an ice cooler stocked with cheese, condiments, vegetables, and your favorite no- or low-carb drinks. (My family likes to stay at motels with "free breakfast," but that too often means the only low-carb offerings are butter and half-n-half coffee creamer.)

Buffets will have several low-carb options for you.

Fast-food restaurants also offer several low-carb options. Order a burger and throw away the bun. Or they may build the burger for you wrapped in lettuce, if you ask. Eat the topping of pizza, not the bread. Fancy salads topped with chicken or beef are commonly available. Nearly all fast-food restaurants provide nutritional analysis for menu items; ask for it if you aren't sure of the carb count.

5. CHEATING

Let's face it: everybody cheats on diets.

It's easier to deal with the truth when you recognize the truth. It's not going to be the end of the world if you go "off plan" for one or two days a year and just eat like everyone else around you. I'm not suggesting pigging out as if you were at a decadent ancient Roman feast. Just eat reasonable amounts of regular, carb-rich foods. You'll probably gain a pound or two (up to a kilogram). Returning to a strict Ketogenic Mediterranean Diet and exercising a little more for a few days will usually resolve the extra weight.

A more common issue is that someone has a craving for a particular food and can't live with the possibility of never eating it again. For instance, I love apple pie and Cinnabon cinnamon rolls; I'd get depressed if I could never again have them. So what I'll do, perhaps every couple months, is have the cinnamon roll (730 calories and 115 grams of carb!) or a large serving of apple pie *instead of a meal.* Call it a "cheat meal." I eat low-carb, maybe even lower than usual, for the remainder of that day. What about eating your usual three daily meals *plus* the cinnamon roll, and just burn off the extra calories with exercise? Sounds logical. But a 150-pound person (68 kg) would need to jump rope for four and a half hours to burn 730 calories. I won't do that, and you won't either.

Cheat days and cheat meals don't work for everyone. Think about alcoholics who have stopped drinking. Standard advice from addiction specialists—and I agree—is that alcoholics should *never* again drink alcohol. Not even a sip. Probably not even non-alcoholic "beer." That's because it's too tempting and could trigger a drinking binge that could be life-threatening. A few people are that way with carbohydrates. You could say they're addicted, or carboholics. They shouldn't have cheat days or cheat meals. Does this apply to you? Only you can answer that.

6. SWEET CRAVINGS

If sweets are your downfall, be aware that cravings tend to dissipate after several months of low-carbing. It may take up to a year. Unfortunately, that doesn't happen for everyone.

If your cravings persist and you can't resist them, your best option is non-caloric artificial sweeteners, sometimes known as sugar substitutes. Examples are sucralose, aspartame, sorbitol, erythritol, and stevia. Several of these can be used in cooking and baking.

Online low-carb recipe repositories will have many sweet options. Or use off-the-shelf prepared items from grocery stores. Try sugar-free gelatin or sugar-free hard candy.

I have no objection if you wish to drink one or two diet soda pops a day. Water may be better for you.

7. HOLIDAYS

Holidays like Thanksgiving (in the U.S.) and Christmas present major temptations to folks trying to limit carb consumption. It's easier to stay "on plan" if you don't socialize much, but most of us visit relatives or others, and the temptation to eat like everyone else is great and often irresistible.

Sometimes people almost "force" carbs on you. Diabetics and prediabetics can say, "No, thanks. My doctor has me on a special diet," and that should be the end of it. Others can say, "I'm fine, thank you. I just feel better if I eat a different way," or, "I'm fine, thank you. I'm not hungry right now." Best of all, say "No, thanks. I'm on Dr. Parker's Ketogenic Mediterranean Diet. It's great. Let me tell you about it!"

Another option is to cheat on the diet.

8. HUNGER

If you get hungry between meals, choose an item from the "unlimited" foods list and see if that helps. Or eat cheese, up to three ounces a day. A can of tuna or a couple hard-boiled eggs may not be your traditional snacks, but they aren't likely to blow your weight management plan compared to a bag of corn chips or handful of cookies.

9. RECORD-KEEPING

You can track your weight, blood sugars, and consumption of the major food items with the "KMD & LCMD Daily Log" available for free at http://advancedmediterraneandiet.com/printabledocuments.html.

If desired, you can pretty easily keep track of your daily consumption online at SELF-NutritionData. The web address is http://nutritiondata.self.com/. First, register your free membership. Then go to the "My ND" section near the top of the page and click on "My Recipes." Make each of your days a single recipe with a title such as "LCMD Day 1." Enter everything you eat in the course of a day. Remember to click "Save" before you leave that day's recipe. At the end of the day, choose the "Save and Analyze" button. You'll get a comprehensive nutritional analysis of that day's consumption.

And I mean *comprehensive*: overall percentages of carbohydrate, protein, and fat, along with total calories and 40 or 50 vitamins, minerals, and other nutrients.

If you're going to do this for more than a couple days, use the "My Foods" feature and you'll end up saving time. An exercise like this—essentially a food diary—over four or five days is also helpful in figuring out why weight loss may have stalled or blood sugars are getting higher. Carb consumption often creeps up unnoticed, and at a certain point will sabotage the best laid plans.

You can do similar record-keeping and nutritional analysis at FitDay (http://fitday.com/). FitDay also helps you easily track your weight and exercise and estimate calories burned exercising. It's definitely worth a look. It's free.

Yet another good free option for record-keeping is Calorie Count (http://caloriecount.about.com/).

Both Calorie Count and FitDay have active community forums for weight-loss support and education.

10. WEIGHT-LOSS TIPS

Record-keeping is often the key to success. For options, see the section immediately preceding this.

Accountability is another key to success. Consider documenting your program and progress on a free website such as FitDay, SparkPeople, 3FatChicks, or others. If your initiation to low-carb eating is a major undertaking (and it should be) consider blogging about your adventure on a free platform such as Wordpress or Blogger. Such a public commitment may be just what you need to keep you motivated.

Do you have a friend or spouse who wants to lose weight? Start the same program at the same time and support each other. That's built-in accountability.

If you tend to over-eat, floss and brush your teeth after you're full. You'll be less likely to go back for more anytime soon.

Eat at least two or three meals daily. Skipping meals may lead to uncontrollable overeating later on. On the other hand, ignore the diet gurus who say you *must* eat every two or three hours.

Eat meals at a leisurely pace, chewing and enjoying each bite thoroughly before swallowing.

Plan to give yourself a specific reward for every 10 pounds (4.5 kg) of weight lost. You know what you like. Consider a weekend get-away, a trip to the beauty salon, jewelry, an evening at the theater, a professional massage, home entertainment equipment, new clothes, etc.

Carefully consider when would be a good time to start your new lifestyle. It should be a period of low or usual stress. Bad times would be Thanksgiving Day, Christmas/New Years' holiday, the first day of a Caribbean cruise, and during a divorce.

If you know you've eaten enough at a meal to satisfy your nutritional requirements yet you still feel hungry, drink a large glass of water and wait a while.

Limit television to less than a few hours a day.

Maintain a consistent eating pattern throughout the week and year.

Eat breakfast routinely.

Control emotional eating.

Weigh frequently: daily during active weight-loss efforts and during the first two months of your maintenance-of-weight-loss phase. After that, cut back to weekly weights if you want. Daily weights will remind you how hard you worked to achieve your goal.

Be aware that you might regain five or 10 pounds (2.3 or 4.5 kg) of fat now and then. You probably will. Don't freak out. It's human nature. You're not a failure; you're human. But draw the line and get back on the old Ketogenic Mediterranean Diet for one or two months. Analyze and learn from the episode. Why did it happen? Slipping back into your old ways? Slacking off on exercise? Too many special occasion feasts or cheat days? Allowing junk food or non-essential carbs back into the house?

Learn which food item is your nemesis: the food that consistently torpedoes your resolve to eat right. For example, mine is anything sweet. Remember an old ad campaign for a potato chip: "Betcha can't eat just one!"? Well, I can't eat just one cookie. So I don't get started. I might eat one if it's the last one available. Or I satisfy my sweet craving with a diet soda, piece of dark chocolate, or sugar-free gelatin. Just as a recovering alcoholic can't drink any alcohol, perhaps you should totally abstain from...? You know your own personal gastronomic Achilles heel. Or heels. Experiment with various strategies for vanquishing your nemesis.

Use a food scale and measuring devices to improve your compliance with portion sizes, especially during the first month. Thereafter you may be able to judge portion size by eye and feel.

One ounce (28 g) of cheese is about the size of a domino.

An ounce (28 g) of nuts is about a quarter of a cup, or a heap of nuts in the palm of your hand, not covering your fingers.

Fish and poultry may be a little more healthful for you than red meat.

Regular meat products may be a little healthier than processed meats like bacon, bologna and other luncheon meats, pre-cooked commercial sausages, etc.

As long as a food is low-carb, don't go for the low-fat version. For instance, low-fat yogurt is over-loaded with carbohydrates compared to the full-fat version.

Tell your housemates you're on a special diet and ask for their support. You may also need to tell your co-workers and others with whom you spend significant time. If they care about you, they'll be careful not to tempt you off the diet.

Do your grocery shopping from a list.

For help with basic culinary skills, peruse these books: How *to Cook Everything: Simple Recipes for Great Food*, by Mark Bittman; *Joy of Cooking: 75th Anniversary Edition*, by Irma S. Rombauer, Marion Rombauer Becker, and Ethan Becker; *Betty Crocker Cookbook: Everything You Need to Know to Cook Today*.

11. SOCIAL ISSUES

AGAINST THE GRAIN OF A CARB-CENTRIC CULTURE

There was a time in my life that I just loved whole grain bread, pizza, and pasta. I couldn't imagine life without them. As an experiment, I went an entire year eating low-carb, without whole grain bread, pizza, and pasta. After that, I didn't miss them much at all. I realized I could easily have a happy, healthy, fulfilling, life without whole grain bread, pizza, and pasta. If you told me I had a medical condition that would worsen if I ate them, I could easily live without them and not complain.

During that same experimental year, I cut way back on my consumption of sweet fruits, starchy vegetables, and sweets (cookies, cakes, candy bars, pies). After the year was up, I didn't miss the sweet fruits and starchy vegetables, although I did miss my sweet things. I could see living the rest of my life without sweet fruits and starchy vegetables. Giving up apple pie and Cinnabon cinnamon rolls would be tougher.

That's just my experience, but I'm not alone. I wouldn't ask you to give up many of your beloved carbohydrates if I didn't know it was possible, and that others had done it successfully. The trade-offs for many of us will be improved health and slimmer waistlines.

The odd thing about the Ketogenic Mediterranean Diets is that it goes against the grain (pun intended) of the Western food culture that prominently features carbohydrates. Anyone following the diet is immediately in a strange position, surrounded continuously with opportunities and inducements to consume carbs. Especially nutrient-depleted, highly refined carbs such as white bread, sugar, flour, fruit juice, potato and corn chips, high fructose corn syrup, and soda pop.

It's difficult to swim against the tide in such a carb-centric culture, especially when you've been enjoying carbs for 30 or 40 years before they finally caused your overweight problem. Old habits are hard to break. Food preferences are deeply ingrained from an early age.

One way to counteract that cultural pull is to take to heart the medical consequences of progressive overweight and obesity as outlined in chapter two. How do you motivate someone today to make a radical change in behavior that may not have a health-related payoff for another decade or more? Education is the only tactic I know that works consistently. People are more receptive when they're hospitalized with diabetic symptoms and blood sugars are 450 mg/dl (25 mmol/l). Even then change is often a struggle.

Low-carb eating increasingly will be seen as viable and healthful as news of recent scientific developments becomes mainstream. Low-carbing will be easier to maintain then, as more folks get on board.

ONLINE SUPPORT

If you feel lonely and odd eating very-low-carb, you'll find copious online support at the Low Carb Friends message boards (http://lowcarbfriends.com/) and Active Low-Carbers Forum (http://forum.lowcarber.org/). There are plenty of low-carbers also on the forums at FitDay, Spark-People, and 3FatChicks.

PARTIES AND HOLIDAY MEALS

In general, I think it's a good idea to let those around you know that you're eating low-carb. I understand there may be good reasons to keep it a secret, however. If you're not in charge of the food, let the host know you'll be focusing on meat, chicken, eggs, fish, cheese, and low-carb vegetables. The meats are usually main courses anyway. You'll simply not be eating many of the side dishes like bread, potatoes, corn, peas, and desserts. If you're the host, I'm sure you'll want to provide your guests—especially children—with the usual high-carb fare. With some experience, you could serve adults a delicious low-carb feast without their awareness.

If the host is a vegetarian or vegan serving his usual cuisine, you may not be able to low-carb. Think about eating before the event, and then just eat a little to be cordial.

7

The Advanced Mediterranean Diet

"**M**ike, your heart's a ticking time bomb." The cardiologist left no room for misinterpretation. 54-year-old Mike was in the hospital with his second heart attack.

The first attack, a mild one, was only a year ago. He didn't have health insurance at the time and wondered if that's why the doctors didn't spend much time with him. He was discharged after five days, with prescriptions for five pills. Aspirin was the only one he could afford. He didn't keep his follow-up appointments out of embarrassment for not being able to pay his doctors and the hospital. The bills from that episode totaled $32,000. At least the healthcare team convinced him to stop his pack-a-day smoking habit, which saved him $5.00 per day, or $1,800 a year. With this second, more serious, heart attack, Mike was motivated to defuse the time bomb.

Mike was a married real estate agent with four kids. He was a TV sports fanatic who enjoyed fishing and flying radio-controlled model airplanes. Earlier in life, he had enjoyed playing baseball and tennis, but he no longer had the interest or energy. Soccer had not been a part of Mike's youth, but he learned enough about it to help coach when two of his kids were players for six years.

Mike met his wife, Susan, when he was 21 and she was 19. After just two or three months of dating, he figured they would be together forever. He kept this thought to himself. Mike had seen too many of his friends mistake infatuation and lust for authentic, enduring love. So they dated for another year before he proposed marriage. Susan was a domestic goddess, i.e., a full-time mommy and homemaker, until the youngest child entered school. Then she returned to the office work force as a secretary. She still did most of the cleaning and cooking. Mike tried to help out, but his concept of "clean" wasn't quite the same as Susan's. As a cook, he couldn't make much more than scrambled eggs, pancakes, and grilled steaks. His specialty was homemade, hand-cranked ice cream. He was an expert microwave button-pusher, but had trouble building peanut butter and jelly sandwiches.

Susan and Mike grew up with, and continued to enjoy, typical Midwestern fare: red meat-centered meals, chicken in all its manifestations, cheesy casseroles, potatoes and corn, bacon and eggs, sausage and biscuits, white bread and butter, and, frequently, dessert. Whole grains and fruits, rarely. His frequent dining out with business associates and clients wasn't any better. Mike enjoyed two or three beers most evenings. And he had a sweet tooth. They rarely ate fish except for an all-U-can-eat fried catfish buffet at a particular restaurant every couple of months.

At the time of his first heart attack, Mike was a classic high-risk heart patient: hypertensive, smoker, sedentary, overweight, diabetic, eating a typical American diet. Diabetes, defined by elevated blood sugars, tends to accelerate the "hardening of the arteries" that causes most heart attacks. The medical term is atherosclerosis. In addition, his "bad cholesterol" was sky high and his "good cholesterol" was in the basement. He had eight risk factors for a heart attack.

Stopping smoking was certainly the best immediate, short-term lifestyle change he could have made to avoid another heart attack. Between his first and second heart attacks, Mike had done nothing new with his diabetes, blood pressure, physical inactivity, cholesterol levels, and excess weight. Luckily, he was able to obtain health insurance just before his second heart attack and was planning to get medical attention. He had the android (apple-shaped) obesity body pattern associated with cardiovascular disease: most of his excess fat was around his waist, with skinny legs and arms. Mike had a 43-inch (109 cm) waistline. At 5-feet, 10-inches (178 cm) tall, weighing 230 pounds (104 kg), his body mass index was an unhealthy 33. A body mass index between 18.5 and 24.9 is optimal for health and longevity.

Early during his second heart attack hospital stay, Mike's cardiologist opened up two heart artery blockages with angioplasty: a balloon in the artery expanded the blocked segment, and metallic stents were left in place to keep the artery open. The cardiologist identified two other areas of 40 and 50% arterial blockage that could cause problems within the next few years, but did not require immediate mechanical intervention. His blood sugars were at their usual too-high levels, 200–300 mg/dl (11–17 mmol/l), compared with nondiabetic levels of 70–140 (3.9–7.8 mmol/l). Sugar levels this high are dangerous in the setting of a fresh heart attack, and over the long run are associated with numerous diabetic complications. I met Mike in the hospital when his cardiologist asked for my help controlling his diabetes. Mike was, indeed, a walking, talking time bomb.

INTRODUCTION

If you just opened this book for the first time and plan on skipping the introduction and chapters one through three, forget it. It won't work. You won't have the necessary knowledge, motivation, and commitment for long-term weight control. No cheating! Begin at the beginning.

After reading chapter four, you may have decided to start with the Ketogenic Mediterranean Diet. The KMD drastically reduces carbohydrate consumption down to 20–40 grams a day, compared to the standard American diet containing 250–300 grams. The theoretical underpinning of the KMD is the carbohydrate/insulin theory or "carbohydrate intolerance" model of overweight and obesity. That is, carbohydrates in our food cause insulin release, which in turn promotes the storage of energy as fat tissue. So to lose weight, you want to reduce insulin action by cutting back on carbs.

But the KMD doesn't suit everybody. That's where the Advanced Mediterranean Diet comes into play. You still lose weight with it even though you're eating more carbohydrates than on the KMD. But you eat fewer carbs than you're eating right now, and you'll be eating better carbs. What are better carbs? The ones that don't lead to dramatic spikes in insulin release. You'll be cutting back in particular on highly refined starches and concentrated sugars (the "fattening carbs"). In reality, both the KMD and AMD acknowledge the carbohydrate/insulin theory; it's just a matter of degree.

It's OK to switch back and forth from KMD to AMD if you wish.

I designed the Advanced Mediterranean Diet for you with three goals in mind:
1. Success in shedding excess fat
2. Success in keeping the weight off
3. Optimization of health and longevity.

Nobody sets out to lose 10, 20, or many more pounds (5, 10, or more kg), and then gain it back without fail. Yet many people unwittingly have done just that. I've done it three or four times. Reasons for failure on many other diets include lack of food variety, excessive regimentation, overwhelming cravings and hunger, weakness and other physical problems, sense of deprivation, expense, difficulty finding ingredients, and food preparation hassle.

A quick glance at Table 5.1 Food Choices and Serving Sizes a few pages forward will lay to rest your concern about variety. Within reasonable boundaries, you decide what and when to eat from that list. The program provides enough fat and protein so you don't have the gnawing hunger suffered so often on low-fat/high-carbohydrate diets. Adequate fiber also contributes to fullness after meals. You won't get physically ill, because I'm giving you adequate calories and all the necessary vitamins, minerals and other micronutrients you need to stay healthy. You'll undoubtedly have to give up some of your favorite things. Maybe your particular nemesis is ice cream, potato chips, cookies, or pie. Alas, they're not on the list. But I give you a diet holiday every two weeks, allowing a return to your guilty pleasure in moderation. The foods on the list are generally no more expensive than what you're already eating. Unlike some diets I've seen, you will not need a personal chef to prepare meals, nor need to live in a multicultural metropolis for access to exotic ingredients.

To lose only five or 10 pounds (2 to 4 kg), you may only need to start a regular exercise program: 30–45 minutes of exercise for five days a week. This works better for men than women. Most people, however, will need to cut back on the number of calories they eat. To make up for the missing calories, your body will convert pounds of stored fat to weightless energy.

TRADITIONAL MEDITERRANEAN DIET DEFINED

What we know today as the healthy Mediterranean diet is based on the Mediterranean diet of the early 1960s, heavily influenced by Greece and southern Italy. It's characterized by small amounts of red meat, less than four eggs per week, low to moderate amounts of poultry and fish, daily fresh fruit, seasonal locally grown foods with minimal processing, concentrated sugars only a few times per week, wine in low to moderate amounts and usually taken at mealtimes, milk products (mainly cheese and yogurt) in low to moderate amounts, olive oil as the predominant fat, and an abundance of food from plants: vegetables, fruits, beans, potatoes, nuts, seeds, breads and other whole grain products.

Ancel Keys was the first prominent scientist to advocate the widespread adoption of the Mediterranean-style diet. His Seven Countries Study was one of the first to associate the Mediterranean diet with improved health. Starting in 1957 and lasting for decades, this study examined relationships between diet and men's health in Italy, Greece, United States, Japan, Finland, the Netherlands, and Yugoslavia. The Mediterranean countries in the Seven Countries Study had lower rates of heart and vascular disease, which Keys attributed to lower blood cholesterol levels and saturated fatty acid intake. Subsequent research failed to confirm the association between cholesterol, saturated fat, and heart disease, but the overall healthiness of the Mediterranean diet has stood the test of time.

Keys lived to be almost 101. He and his biochemist wife, Margaret, popularized the Mediterranean diet over 35 years ago through best-selling books such as *How to Eat Well and Stay Well the Mediterranean Way*.

HEALTH BENEFITS OF THE MEDITERRANEAN DIET

Scientific studies have clearly shown that a Mediterranean-style diet is linked with overall greater health and longevity, lower incidence of cancers (of the colon, breast, prostate, and uterus), lower risk of type 2 diabetes and dementia, and lower rates of cardiovascular disease such as heart attacks and strokes.

Weaker supporting evidence links the Mediterranean diet with slowed progression of dementia, prevention of melanoma (serious skin cancer), lower severity of type 2 diabetes, as judged by diabetic drug usage and blood sugar levels, less risk of developing obesity, better blood pressure control in the elderly, improved weight loss and weight control in type 2 diabetics, improved control of asthma, reduced risk of developing diabetes after a heart attack, reduced risk of mild cognitive impairment, prolonged life of Alzheimer disease patients, lower rates and severity of chronic obstructive pulmonary disease, lower risk of gastric (stomach) cancer, less risk of macular degeneration, less Parkinson's disease, increased chance of pregnancy in women undergoing fertility treatment, reduced prevalence of metabolic syndrome (when supplemented with nuts), lower incidence of asthma and allergy-like symptoms in children of women who followed the Mediterranean diet while pregnant.

Whew! Now you know why the Mediterranean diet is a perennial favorite among dietitians and physicians. No other diet can legitimately claim so many healthful attributes.

The health benefits likely spring from synergy among multiple Mediterranean diet components, rather than from a single food group or one or a few food items.

I've found that nearly everybody's eyes glaze over if I try to explain how, physiologically, the Mediterranean diet promotes health and longevity. For the boring details, see this post at my Diabetic Mediterranean Diet blog:
http://diabeticmediterraneandiet.com/2011/09/02/why-is-the-mediterranean-diet-so-healthy/

WHAT'S WRONG WITH REFINED, PROCESSED FOODS?

The goals of food processing are to increase the attractiveness and marketability of certain foods. Examples of highly processed foods include potato or corn chips, many commercially prepared snacks, regular white flour, sugar-sweetened beverages, candy, ice cream, children's breakfast cereals, and many commercial baked goods. Some of the most well-known foods are highly processed, such as Oreos, Cheetos, and Pop-Tarts, to name a few. Heavily processed, high-carbohydrate foods may be more convenient, less expensive, easier to transport, and may taste great. They often last longer on the shelf.

These attributes have made the modern supermarket possible. But these "easy" foods contribute to our tendency to over-eat. Many lead to heavy release of the fat-building hormone, insulin, from the pancreas

There are other potential drawbacks. Processing may remove or degrade healthful nutrients, and add other substances or nutrients that aren't so healthy. Fresh, minimally processed foods usually have more naturally occurring vitamins, fiber, and minerals (e.g., potassium). Heavily processed foods often have added sugars, fats, sodium, and man-made chemicals that are added for flavor and other reasons, but which can undermine the goal of healthier eating. It's a complex issue. What's clear is that the healthy Mediterraneans of the 1960s were not known for their conspicuous consumption of Twinkies, Doritos, and Froot Loops.

Most overweight people have a major problem with excessive consumption of refined starches and concentrated sugars. It's time to stop eating overprocessed food laden with man-made chemicals and unnatural fats, supercharged with sugar.

ADVANCED MEDITERRANEAN

The composition of your new diet is most succinctly described as Advanced Mediterranean. It maximizes natural, nutrient-dense, whole foods and minimizes highly processed ones. Scientific breakthroughs over the last 15 years have allowed me to fine-tune the traditional Mediterranean diet, likely leading to even greater improvements in health and longevity. Upon review of the scientific literature, I found one hundred and eight eye-opening research reports to support my recommendations, which are built into the program.

WHAT ABOUT WINE?

For centuries, the healthier populations in the Mediterranean region have enjoyed wine in light to moderate amounts, usually with meals. Epidemiologic studies there and in other parts of the world have associated reasonable alcohol consumption with prolonged lifespan, reduced coronary artery disease, diminished Alzheimer's and other dementias, and possibly fewer strokes.

What's a "reasonable" amount of alcohol? An old medical school joke is that a "heavy drinker" is anyone who drinks more than the doctor does. Light to moderate alcohol consumption is generally considered to be one or fewer drinks per day for a woman, two or fewer drinks per day for a man. One drink is 5 ounces (150 ml) of wine, 12 ounces (355 ml) of beer, or 1.5 ounces (45 ml) of 80 proof distilled spirits (e.g., vodka, whiskey, gin). The optimal health-promoting type of alcohol is unclear. I tend to favor wine, a time-honored component of the Mediterranean diet. Red wine in particular is a rich source of resveratrol, which is thought to be a major contributor to the cardioprotective benefits associated with light to moderate alcohol consumption. Grape juice may be just as good—it's too soon to tell.

I have no intention of overselling the benefits of alcohol. If you are considering habitual alcohol as a food, be aware that the health benefits are still somewhat debatable. Consumption of three or more alcoholic drinks per day is clearly associated with a higher risk of breast cancer in women. Even one or two drinks daily may slightly increase the risk. Folic acid supplementation might mitigate the risk. If you are a woman and breast cancer runs in your family, strongly consider abstinence. Be cautious if there are alcoholics in your family; you may have inherited the predisposition. If you take any medications or have chronic medical conditions, check with your personal physician first. For those drinking above light to moderate levels, alcohol is clearly perilous. Higher dosages can cause hypertension, liver disease, heart failure, certain cancers, and other medical problems. And psychosocial problems. And legal problems. And death. Heavy drinkers have higher rates of violent and accidental death. Alcoholism is often fatal.

You should not drink alcohol if you:
- have a history of alcohol abuse or alcoholism
- have liver or pancreas disease
- are pregnant or trying to become pregnant

- may have the need to operate dangerous equipment or machinery, such as an automobile, while under the influence of alcohol
- have a demonstrated inability to limit yourself to acceptable intake levels
- have personal prohibitions due to religious, ethical, or other reasons.

MEDICAL CLEARANCE

Most people try weight-loss programs without the permission and supervision of physicians, and usually without significant adverse effects. However, serious, even life-threatening, medical problems do occasionally crop up. You may have an underlying medical or psychological condition predisposing you to complications. You may even have a treatable illness causing your weight problem. You should consult a physician regarding these matters before beginning any weight-loss program, including this one. Show him or her this book. If you're a type 2 diabetic, consider the Low-Carb Mediterranean Diet (http://diabeticmediterraneandiet.com/low-carb-mediterranean-diet/). If you're pregnant, don't follow the Advanced or Ketogenic Mediterranean Diet for weight loss.

THE PLAN

By now you understand that a successful weight loss effort requires you to eat fewer calories than your body needs to fuel its metabolism and physical activity. Your body will relieve this "fuel deficit" by converting your stored fat to energy. Total starvation, even for just one or two days per week, doesn't work in the long run. You realize also the vital importance of a proper mix of vitamins, minerals, fiber, protein, carbohydrates, and fat in your diet. You're going to eat every day. But what?

My recommendation is that you follow an "exchange diet" that I've formulated to provide you with the optimal combination of nutrients. You choose items to eat from six food groups: grains, vegetables, fruits, fats, milk products, and proteins. See Table 5.1, Food Choices and Serving Sizes. Copy it, attach it to your refrigerator or kitchen cabinet, take a copy to work. Print a copy of it from the AMD website: http://advancedmediterraneandiet.com/printabledocuments.html

Table 5.1 Food Choices and Serving Sizes

Food Choices & Serving Sizes

Grains (100 cal)

1 slice bread, whole grain
¼ cup (60 ml) Post grape-nuts
1 cup (240 ml) Cheerios
½ cup (120 ml) raisin bran
1 oz (30 g) shredded wheat cereal, plain
5 Triscuit Original crackers
3 Ry Krisp Natural crackers
½ cup (120 ml) whole wheat pasta, cooked
½ cup (120 ml) cooked brown rice
1 tortilla, whole grain
½ cup (120 ml) dry oats, whole grain
100 calorie serving of any whole grain breakfast cereal or
         cracker containing at least 3 grams of fiber

Vegetables (60 cal)

1 cup (240 ml) asparagus, green beans, beets, Brussels

149

sprouts, broccoli, carrots, cauliflower, okra, onions, tomatoes, winter squash, canned or boiled spinach
1½ cup (360 ml) summer squash, raw spinach, boiled collard greens, boiled turnip greens, boiled kale, boiled mustard greens
¼ cup (60 ml) cooked dry beans (kidney, pinto, black-eyed peas, lentils, white beans, lima, refried, chickpeas)
10 fl oz (300 ml) vegetable juice
½ sweet potato, medium
2 carrots, medium

2 cups turnips, boiled, cubed   ½ cup (120 ml) green peas
10 olives, green, medium   2 tomatoes, medium
10 olives, black, ripe, medium   1 artichoke, medium
¼ avocado   6 tbsp (90 ml) tomato paste
½ cup (120 ml) water chestnuts 1 cup (240 ml) tomato sauce

Fruits (80 cal)

1 medium apple, banana, orange, pomegranate, peach
1 cup (240 ml) strawberries, blueberries, blackberries, grapes, cubed honeydew or watermelon
½ cup (120 ml) applesauce (unsweetened)
2 tangerines
1/8 cup or 1 oz (30 ml or 30 g) raisins
½ cantaloupe or grapefruit
2 plums, medium

12 cherries, raw   4 dates
½ cup (120 ml) fruit juice   4 oz wine

Fats (110 cal)

1 tbsp (15 ml) oil (esp. olive, canola, flaxseed, soybean)
1-2 tbsp (15-30 ml) salad dressing (read label to get 110 cal)
4 tsp (20 ml) bacon bits
2slices (16 g) pork bacon, cooked
½ oz (15 g) almonds, butternuts, cashews, hazelnuts, macadamia nuts, peanuts, pistachios, soybean nuts, walnuts, pecans, sunflower seeds, pumpkin seeds
1 tbsp (15 ml) mayonnaise
1 tbsp (15 ml) Smart Balance Buttery Spread
1 tbsp (15 ml) butter
2 tbsp (30 ml) Miracle Whip Dressing

2 tbsp (30 ml) cream, heavy
2 tbsp (30 ml) cream cheese

Milk Products (110 cal)

1 oz (30 g) regular cheese
1 cup (240 ml) skim or low-fat milk
¾ cup (180 ml) whole milk
½ cup (120 ml) yogurt, plain, regular, not low-fat
½ cup (120 ml) cottage cheese, regular, not low-fat
4 tbsp (60 ml) grated Parmesan cheese
110 calorie serving of any cheese, milk, or yogurt
(find cream cheese in Fats category)

Proteins (200 cal)

3 ½ oz (100 g) lean beef ("select" or "choice" grade of top round,
      top sirloin, or sirloin tip)
3 ½ oz (100 g) lean (loin/leg) pork, lamb, veal, lean ham
4 oz (110 g) chicken or turkey, light meat, without skin
4 oz (110 g) cold-water fatty fish (e.g., albacore/white tuna,
      herring, mackerel, salmon, sardines, trout, halibut, sea
      bass, swordfish), or other fish if cold-water fatty fish not
      available
¾ cup (180 ml) cooked dry beans (e.g., kidney, pinto, white,
      black-eyed peas, lentils, refried), split peas, chickpeas,
      soybeans, lima beans
1 oz (30 g) almonds, butternuts, cashews, hazelnuts,
      macadamia nuts, peanuts, pistachios, soybean nuts,
      walnuts, pecans, sunflower seeds, pumpkin seeds
4 oz (100 g) buffalo, deer, elk, wild rabbit, ostrich, goat, or
      squirrel
6 oz (170 g) shrimp
6 oz (170 g) lobster
2 tbsp (30 ml) peanut butter
2 chicken eggs, any size
½ cup (120 ml) tofu, raw, firm
1 cup (240 ml) tofu, raw
200 calorie serving of any meat, beef, poultry, fish, pork, lamb,
      or mutton

MAKE IT MEDITERRANEAN!

- Favor fish and poultry over red meat.
- Aim to incorporate 7 to 14 tbsp (100 to 200 ml) olive oil weekly.
- Eat 3 to 5 1-oz (30-g) servings of nuts per week.
- Optional: Drink 4 oz (120 ml) of wine daily.
- Eat at least 2 servings of fish per week.

Table 5.1 Food Choices and Serving Sizes

LET'S GET STARTED!

To see how it works, consider the 1,500 calorie diet (see Table 5.3 1,500 Calorie Daily Log). Although I present other calorie level diets, most active women lose weight nicely and relatively easily eating 1,500 calories daily. On the 1,500 calorie diet, three grain servings are eaten every day. Not two servings, not four, but three. Note the check-off boxes beside "Grains." Look at the listed items under Grains in Table 5.1, Food Choices and Serving Sizes, and eat three of them during every 24 hours, carefully observing portion sizes.

Listed items within a food group in Table 5.1 are roughly equivalent in terms of nutrient mix and calories, and therefore are "exchangeable." This diet also exchanges your body fat for actual usable energy.

1,500 Cal Daily Log   Day:_____
                       Weight:_____

Grains   ☐ ☐ ☐   (100 cal)

Veggies   ☐ ☐   (60 cal)

Fruits   ☐ ☐ ☐   (80 cal)

Fats   ☐ ☐   (110 cal)

Milks   ☐ ☐   (110 cal)

Proteins ☐ ☐   (200 cal)

Exercise:_____

_____

Transgressions:_____

_____

Comments:_____

Table 5.3 1,500 Calorie Daily Log

Perhaps your breakfast includes a slice of whole grain bread. That's one of your three grain servings. Mark it on your Daily Log. Later in the day you eat two more grain servings, marking the log as you go. Do the same for vegetables (two daily check-off boxes in this plan), fruits, fats, milk products, and proteins. When all the boxes are full, you're done eating for the day.

Don't bother to count calories, fat grams, or carbohydrate grams. Photocopy the Daily Log and use a new one every day, noting also your exercise and any inevitable transgressions. Or print your Daily Log by visiting this web page: http://advancedmediterraneandiet.com/printabledo cuments.html

In summary:
1. Determine how much you can eat based on your weight and sex (details later).
2. Check off boxes on a Daily Log as you eat from six food categories.

An alternative to choosing your own food is to follow the easy recipes I provide in chapter nine. You still have to mark off the exchanges as you go, but they're provided with the recipes.

As you can tell from the list of food choices in Table 5.1, this diet has lots of variety. I'm not telling you what to eat every day. I could, but you wouldn't do it for long anyway. You decide what to eat, within broad bounds. If you don't like it, don't eat it.

My eating plan for you doesn't easily allow for "combination foods" such as lasagna, apple pie, soups, or casseroles. Combination foods contain more than one major food item, often in unknown proportions.

When you order lasagna at a restaurant, you may know that it is made from pasta, tomato sauce, meat, and cheese. But you know neither the proportions nor total calorie count of a serving. Therefore, you can't fit it into the exchange diet. Most everybody would underestimate the number of calories on the plate. But you need not forsake combination foods entirely. See item No. 13 under "The Fine Print" later in this chapter.

CHOOSING YOUR CALORIE LEVEL

Now that you understand the plan basics, the next issue is selection of a calorie intake level: 1,100, 1,500, 1,900, or 2,300. This would be easy if you knew how many calories you're eating now to maintain your current steady weight, and how many calories you may burn in a new exercise program.

For example, if we knew that maintenance of your current weight and activity level required 2,000 calories daily, I could tell you to simply reduce your calorie intake to 1,500 daily and you'd lose one pound (454 g) per week. That's because your body still needs 2,000 calories worth of energy and, to get it, will convert 500 calories worth of its fat into energy to go with the 1,500 calories you eat. Recall that a pound (454 g) of fat holds 3,500 calories. Conversion of 500 calories of fat to weightless energy every day for seven days will leave you a pound (454 g) lighter (7 days x 500 calories = 3,500 calories = 1 pound (454 g) of fat in one week).

Alternatively, you could stop eating for two days out of every week and lose a pound (454 g) of fat (2 days x 2,000 calories = 4,000 calories). Would you sign up for that program? I didn't think so. Another way to lose that pound (454 g) would be to keep eating as you are (2,000 calories daily), but increase your physical activity to burn an extra 500 calories daily. The required extra fuel would come from your fat tissue. Few people, however, would tolerate or comply with this marked increase in daily activity. That's why I recommend a combination of moderate reduction in caloric intake and moderate increase in exercise to achieve that daily 500 calorie deficit. In the ideal world, to lose a pound per week I'd like to see you cut daily food intake by 200–300 calories and increase your activity level by 200–300 calories.

In the real world, selection of your Advanced Mediterranean Diet calorie level comes down to flexible "educated guesstimates" and rules-of-thumb. So here goes:

- Overweight women between 130 and 210 pounds (60 to 95 kg) start with the 1,500 calorie plan.
- Women 210 to 300 pounds (95 to 136 kg) start with 1,900 calories.
- Overweight men between 150 and 220 pounds (68 to 100 kg) start with the 1,900 calorie diet.
- Men 220 to 350 pounds (100 to 159 kg) use the 2,300 calorie plan.

Women over 300 (136 kg) and men over 350 pounds (159 kg) infrequently have success with self-help methods such as this book, but are free to try the 2,300 calorie diet with my sincere best wishes. See Tables 5.2 through 5.5 for the various calorie level Daily Logs.

1,100 Cal Daily Log   Day:_____
                        Weight:____

Grains   ☐ ☐   (100 cal)

Veggies   ☐ ☐   (60 cal)

Fruits   ☐ ☐ ☐   (80 cal)

Fats   ☐   (110 cal)

Milks   ☐ ☐   (110 cal)

Proteins   ☐   (200 cal)

Exercise:_____

_____

Transgressions:_____

_____

Comments:_____

Table 5.2 1,100 Calorie Daily Log

```
1,900 Cal Daily Log     Date:_____
                        Weight:____

Grains      □ □ □ □      100 cal)

Veggies     □ □ □        (60 cal)

Fruits      □ □ □ □      (80 cal)

Fats        □ □ □       (110 cal)

Milks       □ □         (110 cal)

Proteins    □ □         (200 cal)

Exercise:_____

        _____

Transgressions:_____

        _____

Comments:_____
```

Table 5.4 1,900 Calorie Daily Log

2,300 Cal Daily Log   Date:_____
                       Weight:____

Grains   ☐ ☐ ☐ ☐ ☐   (100 cal)

Veggies   ☐ ☐ ☐ ☐   (60 cal)

Fruits   ☐ ☐ ☐ ☐   (80 cal)

Fats   ☐ ☐ ☐   (110 cal)

Milks   ☐ ☐ ☐   (110 cal)

Proteins ☐ ☐ ☐   (200 cal)

Exercise: _____

_____

Transgressions: _____

_____

Comments: _____

Table 5.5 2,300 Calorie Daily Log

WHAT IF I'M NOT GOING TO EXERCISE?

The preceding calorie level guidelines are formulated to yield a weekly weight loss of one or one-and-a-half pounds when the diet is followed in conjunction with a light to moderate exercise program. If you're unable or unwilling to exercise regularly, go to the next lower calorie level and start there.

REASSESS CALORIE LEVEL AFTER 1 OR 2 WEEKS

I cannot guarantee that *you* will lose one or one-and-a-half pounds (about half a kg) per week, but the average person will. One-half pound (¼ kg) in some weeks, two pounds (1 kg) in others. Determine your baseline weight, try the recommended calorie intake level for one or two weeks, then re-weigh yourself. Take further action based on your weight outcome:

1. If you lost an average of one to one-and-a-half pounds (about half a kg) per week: Congratulations! You nailed it! Continue your program.

2. If you lost more than one-and-a-half or two pounds (about a kg) per week on average: Great! But be aware much of this loss may be intestinal contents or water, not fat. Continue your current program only if you feel good, optimistic, and not particularly deprived of food. If not, go to the next higher calorie level (for example, from 1,500 to 1,900) and try it for one or two weeks, then re-assess, etc.

3. If your weight held steady or you gained a little or lost less than a pound (half a kg) per week on average: Go to the next lower calorie level and try it for one or two weeks. For example, you started at the 1,500 calorie level, your weight didn't budge, so move to the

1,100 calorie diet for one or two weeks then reassess, etc.

REASONABLE EXPECTATIONS

Many people lose three to five pounds (1.4 to 2.3 kg) in the first week or two of the program. If you're one of the lucky ones, enjoy it, brag about it! Tell all your friends about this wonderful Advanced Mediterranean Diet! But that rate of loss will not be sustainable or safe for more than a couple weeks. And most of the loss isn't fat. Forget about the grandiose claims of other weight loss plans. If you lose over two pounds (1 kg) per week on my program, averaged over three to four weeks, you're losing too fast and need to go to the next higher calorie level. Otherwise you're at risk for medical complications (from nutrient deficiencies) and diet burnout ("I can't stand this anymore. I quit!")

I cannot tell you with precision the calorie intake level that will lead to your loss of one pound per week. Two "wild cards" control the game: 1) your individual basal metabolic rate (BMR), and 2) your individual calorie-burning rate during physical activity. Two people may play a game of tennis, but one of them can burn twice as many calories as the other! BMR is determined predominantly by age, sex, amount of body fat, and lean body mass (e.g., amount of muscle tissue). But BMR varies significantly among individuals who otherwise appear similar. For example, consider two 165-pound (75 kg) women with identical activity levels, neither gaining nor losing weight: One woman is living on 1,600 calories per day, the other requires 2,400. The 2,400-calorie lady gets to eat more food, yet doesn't gain weight. It may not be fair, but that's the way it is.

If you're interested in an estimate of your current weight-stable calorie consumption, try the web-based calculator at: http://advancedmediterraneandiet.com/dailyenergy calculator.html

You could estimate your current calorie intake there, then choose a diet calorie level about 500 calories lower. With luck, you'd lose about a pound (half a kg) per week, plus more if you exercised. But no calculator can account for the mysterious variation in basal metabolic rate between individuals who otherwise look identical.

As you can see, we're trying to find a calorie intake level that, combined with physical activity, will yield one to one-and-a-half pounds of fat loss weekly. This necessarily involves a bit of trial and error. If you were losing a pound per week but wanted to lose one-and-a-half, you could either reduce caloric intake further or burn more calories on physical activity. In the short-term, it makes little difference if you choose "more exercise" over "cutting calories" further. But most people find it much easier to skip that 250-calorie candy bar than to jog an extra 30 minutes on the treadmill.

Most people who have reduced their salt intake to help control high blood pressure eventually find they prefer low-salt eating. It may take a couple months. A similar phenomenon happens with Advanced Mediterranean eating. It will take at least eight to 12 weeks of practice to alter your preference for your old way of eating. Don't give up early.

I advocate weight loss of about a pound (half a kg) per week, or two pounds (1 kg) at most, mainly because it works over the long run. It's sustainable and safe. The weight lost is indeed fat tissue. Other programs tout losses of three to five pounds per week, but much of that loss is water, muscle protein, or intestinal contents. Your body cannot tolerate this for long and will work against your mind to repair or limit the physiologic damage.

A reasonable rate-of-weight-loss goal also will limit the sense of sacrifice and deprivation that torpedoes so many diets. Even on my diet, there will be times when you feel food deprivation, usually mild and transient. Hey, I never said it was easy! Never forget at those times, when you're most hungry, that's when your body is burning fat. You're instantaneously losing weight.

If persistent nagging hunger is a problem, try the Ketogenic Mediterranean Diet in chapter five.

CAN I TAKE A BREAK, DOC?

On your journey toward a personal realistic or healthy weight, you may well need a few rest stops. Consider following the diet carefully for six weeks, stopping for two weeks, then resuming for six weeks, etc. The pause may be refreshing. During the two-week hiatus, continue your exercise program and eat the same basic cuisine as on the diet. You should be able to increase your daily calories by 200–400 and yet hold steady on your overall weight. If you're concerned you'll overeat during the hiatus, simply jump up to the next higher calorie diet. For instance, if you're on the 1,500 calorie plan and steadily losing a pound (half a kg) per week, go up to the 1,900 plan for a two-week break. This strategy particularly appeals to my patients who have slowly gained 50-plus pounds (23-plus kg) of fat over 10 to 15 years. The thought of "being on a diet" continuously for a year is daunting. In reality, for many such people the diet starts to become second nature after a couple months of adherence. It's much less hassle; e.g., minimal measurement of food portions.

WEIGHT-LOSS STALL

After a month or two on a given calorie level diet, and particularly as you near your weight loss goal, you may notice a diminishing return for your honest effort. For instance, you may be cruising along at one-and-a-half pounds (¾ kg) average weekly weight loss, then mysteriously find the weight loss rate dropping to one-half pound (¼ kg) per week or you stop losing weight altogether. This is normal. It's fairly predictable after the loss of 30 to 40 pounds (14 to 18 kg). I'll skip the physiologic explanation this time. Rest assured, you'll get back on track if you cut down to the next lower calorie intake level or increase the duration or intensity of your physical workouts.

WEIGHTS AND MEASURES

Get an accurate scale for weighing yourself. Weigh yourself first thing in the morning, every morning, naked, and after urinating. Keep a written record. Two or three consecutive morning weights will give you a truer picture than one morning. If you have a scale that is a little different every time you step on it, take three readings and record the average. These early morning weights are the most consistent and reliable. It's typical for a person's weight to vary over a range of one to four pounds (0.5 to 1.8 kg) during 24 hours, depending on fullness of the bladder and intestines, state of hydration, time since last meal, etc. If you work nights, weigh yourself in this fashion after you've had your seven to eight hours of sleep. The ritual of daily weighing is partly to keep you honest and compliant with the diet. It's a reminder that you're still on a diet. Furthermore, because of the variability of your weight over the course of a day, it takes three to four days to see a clear, reliable trend.

Women with childbearing potential may need a reminder that some women routinely gain an extra two to four pounds (1 kg) of fluid during the week prior to menstrual bleeding. When assessing your weight change, be sure to take this into account and not overreact if "it's that time of the month."

Record a baseline measurement of your circumference at the chest, waist, and hips. Measure your height and determine your body mass index. Check your resting heart rate and blood pressure. Re-measure periodically, perhaps every two months. Keep a written record for comparison.

After your read "The Fine Print" and "Practical Pearls" you can get started! Don't skip chapter 11, which discusses prevention of weight regain after your months of effort pay off. Godspeed!

THE FINE PRINT

1. Record-keeping is critical. Keep a daily log. Design your own or photocopy the samples I provide. Note 1) your compliance with food group servings, 2) any transgressions, 3) anything that may have precipitated transgressions, 4) a description of exercise done, 5) daily weight, 6) anything else you deem pertinent. Note changes in blood lipids if pertinent.

2. I recommend regular exercise. More on this later.

3. Plan on grocery shopping, meal preparation, and taking meals to your workplace.

4. Use a food scale and measuring devices to monitor portion sizes, especially during the first few weeks. Just how much *is* an ounce (30 g) of cheese or 3.5 ounces (100 g) of beef or a half ounce (15 g) of nuts? Three ounces (85 g) of cooked beef, chicken, or fish is about the size of a deck of playing cards. One ounce (30 g) of cheese is about the size of a domino. A half cup (120 ml) of cooked pasta is about the same volume as half a baseball.

5. Observe the prescribed number of servings within each food group. If and when you deviate from the food group allocations, at least honor the total calorie limit.

6. Take a multivitamin/multimineral supplement daily, "just to be sure." I like Centrum. Also take enough extra vitamin D to hit 800–1,200 IU daily. Note that your multivitamin may come with 400 IU vitamin D. Also consider supplementing with calcium, 500–1,000 mg of elemental calcium per day. Among other things, vitamin D helps your body use the calcium, which is particularly important in prevention of osteoporosis. Tums is an inexpensive source of calcium. Citracal is another good source. Calcium supplementation is controversial; some experts think it may not be necessary. It's more likely to be beneficial to women than to men. Talk to your personal physician.

7. Eat fish at least twice per week, favoring the cold-water, fatty fish. If you don't, consider taking a fish oil supplement of 1,000 milligrams omega-3 fatty acids daily. The richest fish sources of the healthy omega-3 fatty acids (DHA and EPA) are al-

bacore (white) tuna, salmon, sardines, trout, sea bass, swordfish, herring, mackerel, anchovy, halibut, and pompano. If you're pregnant, trying to become pregnant, or a nursing mother, avoid eating king mackerel, swordfish, shark, and tilefish (sold as golden snapper or golden bass). These fish may contain amounts of mercury harmful to breast-fed infants and babies in the womb.

8.   Unless otherwise specified, listed portion sizes refer to prepared, cooked food without bones.

9.   You may use two or three tablespoons (30 or 45 ml) daily of condiments such as picante sauce, ketchup, or "lite" pancake syrup. Jam, jelly, and honey should be limited to one or two teaspoons (five or 10 ml) daily. One teaspoon (5 ml) of sugar daily is acceptable (15 calories).

10.   You may have these daily bonus foods in addition to other prescribed items, if desired: three celery stalks and one cup (240 ml) zucchini, radishes, mushrooms, or cucumbers, *and* two cups (480 ml) lettuce, *and* 1 cup (240 ml) parsley. *Or* one sweet pepper. *Or* 3 tbsp (45 ml) diced green chiles.

11.   Wine is the only form of alcohol on the diet; 4 oz (120 ml) is listed as a fruit choice and has 80 calories. Limit wine to 4 oz (120 ml) per day. Be aware that 12 oz (355 ml) of beer has 150 calories and distilled spirits have 100–125 calories per 1.5 oz (4.4 ml) jigger.

12.   Eat at least three to five 1-ounce (30 g) servings of nuts weekly. An ounce (30 g) of nuts is not much, about a quarter of a cup (60 ml).

13.   Although it is perhaps best to avoid combination foods such as casseroles and soups, you may

on occasion fit them into the plan. Pay close attention to total calories and try to allocate those calories to the correct food group. For example, frozen Stouffer's Lasagna with Meat and Sauce has 330 calories per one cup (240 ml) serving, according to the box. Listed ingredients, in order, are tomato puree, macaroni (from wheat), cheese, then beef, etc. No amounts are given. You estimate that your cup (240 ml) of lasagna has one of our grain servings (100 cal), one vegetable serving (60 cal of tomato), and one serving of cheese (110 cal). Your diet's meat serving size is 3.5 oz (100 g) beef, which has 200 calories, but you figure the lasagna only has about half that amount (100 cal) in a cup (240 ml). So measure your one cup (240 ml) serving, then mark on your Daily Log one grain, one veggie, one milk product, and a half meat exchange. That's 100 + 60 + 110 + 100 = 370 calories. You can also easily accommodate combination foods if you follow a recipe with known ingredient amounts and calories per serving. For example, see the recipes in chapter nine for some combination foods I've analyzed and recommend to you.

14. Eat a variety of foods within each of the six food groups. This ensures you get all the necessary micronutrients.

15. Each day, you may substitute one-half cup (120 ml) cooked beans for a grain. Check them off as a grain serving.

16. Every two weeks reward yourself with a reasonable evening meal of your choice, disregarding the diet. No pigging out!

17. Avoid substituting with non-listed foods, particularly highly-processed items. But if you do, and you probably will, carefully account for the calories

on your daily log. For example, 8 oz (240 ml) of Co-ca-Cola has 100 calories. Check off a 100 or 110 calorie box.

18. Favor fish and poultry over red meat.

PRACTICAL PEARLS

1. Tell your housemates you're on a diet and ask for their support. You may also need to tell your co-workers and others with whom you spend significant time. If they care about you, they will be careful not to tempt you off the diet.

2. If a food item isn't on the list of food choices, don't keep it in the house unless you're sure it won't tempt you beyond your limits.

3. Eat at least three meals daily. Skipping meals may lead to uncontrollable overeating later on.

4. Learn about spices and other seasonings as flavor substitutes for fats and sugars. Seasonings have few, if any, calories; use ad lib. Prominent Mediterranean spices are cumin, paprika, turmeric, cinnamon, ginger, coriander, anise, Spanish saffron, lemon, mint, parsley, garlic, dill, pepper, and sumac. It's unknown whether these contribute to the life-prolonging and disease-preventing qualities of the Mediterranean diet.

5. While losing weight, use relatively low-fat cooking methods for meat and vegetables: bake, grill, steam, broil, boil, sauté lightly, microwave. Consider nonstick cooking spray, such as PAM. Deep-fat frying is forbidden since you won't know how many calories are in the serving.

6. To satisfy sweet cravings, use sugar-free gelatin, sugar-free hard candy, or diet soda pop.

7. If unplanned snacking after meals is a problem for you, flossing and brushing your teeth right after meals may strengthen your resolve.

8. Do your grocery shopping from a list. Check out this link for a printable AMD grocery shopping list: http://advancedmediterraneandiet.com/printabledo cuments.html

9. Store food out of sight. Out of sight, out of mind. Keep all food in the kitchen.

10. If meals don't give you a full, satisfied feeling, try drinking a full glass of water before meals. Also try a sugar-free psyllium fiber supplement such as Metamucil (3 grams of fiber per rounded teaspoon or 5 ml) with 8 ounces (240 ml) of water around meal time.

11. Eat meals at a leisurely pace, chewing and enjoying each bite thoroughly before swallowing. Traditional Mediterranean meals are a time for socializing, too.

12. Plan to give yourself a specific reward for every 10 pounds (4.5 kg) of weight lost. You know what you like. Consider a weekend get-away, a trip to the beauty salon, jewelry, an evening at the theater, a professional massage, home entertainment equipment, new clothes, etc.

13. Carefully consider when would be a good time to start your new lifestyle. It should be a period of low or usual stress. Bad times would be Thanksgiving Day, Christmas/New Years holiday, the first day of a Caribbean cruise, and during a divorce.

14. For at least a few times, try presenting your food on attractive dishes with a decorative place mat. Eat slowly to allow yourself time to enjoy your food and to appreciate when you're full.

15. For help with basic culinary skills plus hundreds of adaptable recipes, peruse these cookbooks: *How to Cook Everything: Simple Recipes for Great Food*, by Mark Bittman; *Joy of Cooking: 75th Anniversary Edition*, by Irma S. Rombauer, Marion Rombauer Becker, and Ethan Becker; *Betty Crocker Cookbook: Everything You Need to Know To Cook Today*; and *The New Best Recipes*, by the editors of Cook's Illustrated magazine. On the Internet, see http://www.allrecipes.com or http://www.recipezaar.com for thousands of recipes, plus detailed nutritional analyses.

16. For information on Mediterranean-style cuisine and specific recipes, these books are good sources: *The Mediterranean Diet*, by Marissa Cloutier, M.S., R.D., and Eve Adamson; *The Essential Mediterranean: How Regional Cooks Transform Key Ingredients Into the World's Favorite Cuisines*, by Nancy Harmon Jenkins; *The Mediterranean Kitchen*, by Joyce Goldstein; *Mediterranean Cooking*, by Paula Wolfert; *The New Mediterranean Diet Cookbook: A Delicious Alternative for Lifelong Health*, by Nancy Harmon Jenkins; *The Mediterranean Heart Diet*, by Helen V. Fisher with Cynthia Thomson, Ph.D., R.D.; and *Eat, Drink, and Be Healthy*, by Walter C. Willett, M.D. Recipes in the latter three books include detailed nutritional analysis and calories per serving, which is quite helpful when you incorporate these recipes into the Advanced Mediterranean Diet. On the Internet, check out http://www.gourmed.com, www.allrecipes.com, and www.videojug.com.

17. Gnawing hunger is infrequent with the Advanced Mediterranean program. It may be a sign that you're exercising excessively. Try cutting back on physical activity, and accept a slower rate of weight loss. Or try the Ketogenic Mediterranean Diet.

FOOD GROUPS

Now let's learn more about the various food groups on the Food Choices and Serving Size list, and how to incorporate them into a healthy diet.

GRAINS

Grains are a straightforward food category on the Food Choices list. A grain serving has about 100 calories and 2.5 or more grams of fiber. Maximize whole grain products. Grains often work well at any meal throughout the day, and as snacks.

When looking to add whole grain foods to your diet, read food packages carefully. The name of the product may be misleading: "multigrain" and "seven-grain" breads may not be primarily whole grain. Just because it's brown doesn't mean the bread is whole grain. Read the ingredient list and look for whole grain or whole wheat as the first ingredient, not enriched flour. Other key first ingredients are oats, corn, quinoa, spelt, barley, buckwheat, kamut, amaranth, or kasha.

Acceptable choices will have at least 2.5 grams of fiber per 100 calories. Savvy marketers are increasingly using "whole grain" in product labeling to attract smart, nutrition-conscious consumers. When you find a whole grain product meeting these criteria, you may substitute 100 calories of it for the grains I designate in the "Food Choices and Serving Sizes" list.

Some of the chain Italian restaurants are beginning to offer whole wheat pasta instead of the standard refined wheat product, if you ask. Unlike 10 years ago, your local supermarket probably offers whole wheat pasta now. Watch out for whole wheat "blend" pasta made primarily from standard refined, enriched flour to which they added back fiber removed in the refining process. Look for "whole wheat" as the first ingredient. In choosing whole grain crackers off the shelf, try to avoid trans fats that are added to prolong shelf life.

VEGETABLES

A veggie serving in my scheme is about 60 calories, which is twice the size of a vegetable serving specified by many others, equaling two servings in terms of cancer prevention.

Legumes, which are relatively packed with calories, are included here although they are not technically vegetables. So while a cup of green beans is a generous serving, a quarter cup of cooked dry beans is a bit skimpy in my estimation. But the servings of each have the same number of calories. OK, so I had to do some pigeonholing to make this whole thing work. But it's for your own good.

Measure serving sizes for the first month or so of the diet so you learn what volume of your favorite veggies is 60 calories. It's easy to accidentally overeat calorie-dense items such as beans, avocados, and peas. The widespread tendency to overeat certain vegetables is why you don't see corn and white potatoes on the list. You can add them later after you lose your excess weight.

Go for fresh vegetables to maximize flavor and perhaps nutrient content. They will be less expensive in season and locally grown. Check your local farmers' market. Frozen and canned vegetables are also good for you! Don't worry about the salt in canned vegetables raising your blood pressure; weight loss and exercise will lower your pressure.

The challenge sometimes with vegetables is to make them tasty. Consult your cookbooks or the recipes in chapter nine. The "problem" of seasoning veggies is an opportunity to use olive oil and other beneficial fats. Add zing to many veggies by sautéing in butter, Smart Balance Buttery Spread, or the ever-popular olive oil and garlic. Or coat vegetables cooked other ways with these and other seasonings. Don't forget salt and pepper. Watch out for frozen veggies packaged with buttery or other sauces that add unexpected calories; note the calorie count and portion size provided by the maker.

When you eat beans from a can, beware ingredients that add stealth calories from sugar or fat: baked beans are notorious. Read the label.

FRUITS

Fruits are easy to incorporate into your new lifestyle. A fruit serving has approximately 80 calories. Try fruits you never had before. Buy local and in season to save money. When fresh fruit is unaffordable, unappealing, or inconvenient, there are always raisins and applesauce. Secondarily, resort to canned, dried, or frozen fruit. Watch out for added sugar in canned fruit. Whole fruit is much preferable to store-bought fruit juice; with commercial juices you often lose fiber and gain pure sugar and man-made chemicals.

FATS

A fat serving is about 110 calories. Oils are fats that are liquid at room temperature. The particularly healthy oils are olive, canola, flaxseed, and soybean. Especially olive oil.

Aim to incorporate 7 to 14 tbsp (100 to 200 ml) of olive oil weekly: closer to 7 tbsp (100 ml) if on the 1,100 or 1,500 calorie diet, closer to 14 tbsp (200 ml) if on the 1,900 or 2,300 calorie level. Consider using it to sauté vegetables, as salad dressing, drizzled over pasta, or dip bread in it. It should replace many of the fats in your old diet.

You may think it odd that nuts are included as fats, but 70% of nut calories are from fats. You could use one or two of your fat servings as a nut snack.

You'll find many of the healthy oils on the Food Choices list in store-bought salad dressings. Or make your own vinegar and olive oil dressing; it's not hard. Chapter eight has some great olive oil vinaigrette recipes. Measure, then pour over your raw vegetables, including the "bonus foods" mentioned in the Fine Print (celery, zucchini, radishes, cucumbers, lettuce).

Did I mention sautéing with olive oil and garlic? Delicious!

MILK PRODUCTS

These items are notable for calcium, high-quality protein, vitamin D, riboflavin, potassium, magnesium, and fat. A milk product serving has 110 calories. The list includes whole milk and regular cheese as well as low-fat milk, yogurt, and cottage cheese.

These items are pretty straightforward in terms of incorporation into your diet. Eat them by themselves or add milk to your whole grain breakfast cereal. Add Parmesan or other cheeses to vegetable dishes and salads. Top bread or crackers with cheese.

The low-fat versions of milk products too often substitute carbohydrates for the fat that was removed, often with little or no savings in terms of total calories. Yogurt is notorious for this. When the Mediterraneans of the 1950s and 1960s ingested yogurt, cheese, and milk, it was all standard fat content; "reduced fat," "low fat," and "fat free," items hadn't been developed yet. Low-fat versions were developed out of concern that dietary total fat and saturated fat caused heart and vascular disease. Now that we know that's not the case, I prefer the regular, full-fat versions for myself. The added carbohydrates in the low- and no-fat versions may actually contribute to overweight.

Flavor your plain yogurt with fresh fruit or non-caloric syrups from DaVinci or other sources.

If you have lactose intolerance—inability to digest milk products—you may yet be able to digest yogurt, cottage cheese, hard cheeses, and acidophilus milk. Another option is to add lactase enzyme drops or tablets to milk. Some milk products are available pre-treated with the enzyme you lack. Even without added lactase, many lactose-intolerant people can tolerate up to two cups of milk daily if it's taken with meals and spread throughout the day.

If none of this appeals to you, simply replace the milk product calories (110 per serving) with anything else on the list of food choices, replacing calorie for calorie. Diets without milk products may be deficient in calcium, so consider a daily elemental calcium supplement of 500 or 1,000 mg along with 800–1,200 IU of vitamin D. Milk products are also a major source of riboflavin; be sure your multivitamin has it.

PROTEINS

The protein servings have about 200 calories. Food derived from animals provides us with copious protein of high quality, usually accompanied by some fat. We need the amino acids in these proteins so we can produce and repair our body's various tissues and enzymes.

Vegetarians can obtain the same amino acids by eating the proper mix of plants. Certain plants have much more protein than others, so you can eat these as alternatives to animals and still obtain the amino acids your body needs to be healthy. Examples are legumes, nuts, and tofu (made from soybeans). If you regularly eat beans as a substitute for meat, chicken, and fish, you should eat them with grains in a ratio of approximately one part beans to three parts grains. This will ensure adequate amino acids to build the proteins your body needs.

Two items in this list may be particularly beneficial in terms of heart health: fish and nuts. Eat at least two servings of fish per week, preferably the cold-water, fatty fish. The richest fish sources of the healthy omega-3 fatty acids (DHA and EPA) are albacore (white) tuna, salmon, sardines, trout, sea bass, swordfish, herring, mackerel, anchovy, halibut, and pompano. If fish seems too expensive or inconvenient, consider canned sardines, tuna, or kippered herring.

Aim to eat three to five 1-ounce (30-g) servings of nuts per week. It's easy to eat too many nuts, sabotaging your weight-loss effort. If you have this problem, measure out the proper amount (1 ounce or 30 g), then close and put away the main jar or bag. If you have trouble stopping nut consumption once you get started, put your dose in a baggie and eat them at work or away from home, so you can't easily return to the mother lode. Or have a housemate hide them!

Consumption of fish and nuts is especially important if you have a personal or family history of heart disease, such as heart attacks.

One caveat concerning fish consumption is that fish may contain harmful chemical contaminants, such as mercury (also known as methylmercury), dioxins, and polychlorinated biphenyls. Methylmercury tends to accumulate in the tissues of some species, especially larger, predatory fish. Methylmercury can potentially disrupt the development of the nervous system in fetuses and infants. But for most people, the potential benefits of moderate fish consumption far outweigh the potential risks of various contaminants. However, if you're pregnant, trying to become pregnant, or a nursing mother, avoid eating king mackerel, swordfish, shark, and tilefish (sold as golden snapper or golden bass). These fish may contain amounts of mercury harmful to breast-fed infants and babies in the womb. On the other hand, at least one scientific study suggests that low seafood intake during pregnancy impairs optimal brain development of children. Healthy seafood components, such as omega-3 fatty acids, may be very beneficial to nervous system growth of the baby in the womb. To complicate things further, not all tuna are created equal. Albacore (white) tuna is a good source of the healthy omega-3 fatty acids, but tends to have three times higher mercury levels than "light tuna," which has much less omega-3s. Fish oil capsules, on the other hand, contain no mercury.

If you eat lots of locally caught freshwater fish, especially if you are a woman of childbearing age, check with your regional governmental authorities regarding contaminants. In the United States, the appropriate state agency is usually the Health Department or Game and Fish Department. Please don't reject fish consumption altogether as too risky and confusing. Adult medical problems attributable to chemical fish contamination are exceedingly rare.

Many of the protein foods can be grilled, sautéed, baked, or added to soups. Use some of your fat servings by marinating fish, poultry, pork, or red meat in store-bought zesty Italian salad dressing before grilling. If you purchase canned meats or fish, get the kind packed in water, not oil; that way the calories are easier to track.

Eggs are a cheap source of quality proteins and certain vitamins. Experts have been debating for the last 40 years whether dietary cholesterol in eggs is harmful in terms of vascular health. The jury is still out, but my sense is that it's not much of a problem. Cardiovascular risk of egg consumption is probably minimal or nonexistent for anyone eating Advanced Mediterranean-style, starting a lifelong exercise program, and permanently losing 50 or more pounds (23-plus kg) of excess weight. If you or your physician are concerned, limit eggs to four to seven per week. "Everything in moderation" applies here.

MIKE'S EPILOGUE

Now back to Mike's story, from the beginning of this chapter. He was the 54-year-old walking, talking, time bomb with numerous risk factors for future heart attacks: high blood pressure, obesity, diabetes, adverse cholesterols, smoking, sedentary lifestyle, typical American diet, and age. Many of these issues also increased his odds of suffering strokes or cancer. Remember, heart attacks, strokes, and cancer are the top three causes of death in the United States. Not to mention disability. We can't stop the aging process, but all of Mike's other risk factors were modifiable. Mike quit smoking of his own volition, for which he has my respect. But without additional intervention, Mike's future was not bright. I convinced Mike that the Advanced Mediterranean Diet program was the way to defuse the bomb. (I treated Mike before developing the Ketogenic Mediterranean Diet, which is probably even better for diabetics.) I gave him the tools, but he had to wield them himself.

Mike already knew how to cook over-processed flour pancakes, so it was natural for him to experiment with various whole grain pancake recipes. Fishing was one of his hobbies, so he learned how to catch and cook trout, adding Trout Amandine to his list of cooking specialties. He learned why baked fish was more healthful than breaded, deep-fried catfish. Since he "brown-bagged" his work lunches, he took tuna fish sandwiches at least once per week. He found a few wines to substitute for his beer. He ate nuts and fruit in place of his previous potato chip snacks. His wife, Susan, came on board by learning new ways to cook a variety of vegetables, meat, and cold-water, fatty fish. She replaced highly refined grain products with whole grains. After all, like Mike, she wanted the two of them to be "together forever."

Mike started a daily walking program with the blessings of his cardiologist. After he lost about 30 pounds (14 kg) and was more physically fit, he took up tennis again. He started with doubles tennis since that was easier than singles. Eventually, he was in good enough shape to hike to some secluded, wilderness lakes that held ginormous trout. Many other fishermen were too fat and out-of-shape to get there.

Mike weighed 230 pounds (105 kg) and had a body mass index of 33 when I met him. He reduced his weight to the 180–185 (83 kg) range and stabilized there, with a body mass index of 26. Not perfect, but much healthier than a BMI of 33. He worked closely with his primary care physician and consulting endocrinologist on good diabetes control. His exercise and weight loss program enabled him to stop one of his two diabetic pills. He was also able to stop a blood pressure drug and a cholesterol-lowering pill. When he left the hospital Mike was on seven different drugs; a year later, only four. More importantly, he felt better and had considerably rosier medical prospects. Mike took charge of his modifiable risk factors. He defused the bomb.

WHAT ARE YOU WAITING FOR? GET STARTED!

See chapter 10 regarding the role of exercise in weight loss, prevention of weight regain, and for health benefits. Don't miss chapter 11 for long-term maintenance of weight loss.

KEY POINTS

- Observe portion sizes.
- Favor natural, whole foods over highly processed items.
- Your new diet has plenty of variety. Enjoy it. Try new foods.
- A Mediterranean-style diet is associated with greater health and longevity, lower incidence of cancer, less dementia, and lower incidence of cardiovascular disease.
- The predominant source of fat in the Mediterranean diet is olive oil, which is rich in monounsaturated fatty acids.
- People with high consumption of nuts have fewer fatal heart attacks. Eat at least three to five 1-ounce (30-gram) servings of nuts weekly.
- Liberal intake of cold-water, fatty fish protects against heart disease, perhaps as a result of omega-3 polyunsaturated fatty acids. Eat fish at least twice per week.
- Reasonable alcohol consumption is associated with prolonged lifespan, reduced coronary artery disease, and diminished Alzheimer's and other dementias.
- Legumes may reduce the risk of coronary heart disease. Aim for four servings per week.
- Aim for weight loss of 1 to 1½ pounds (½ to ¾ kg) per week.

- Record-keeping is critical. Keep a daily log of food intake and exercise. Weigh daily until you reach your goal, then weekly.
- Regular physical activity is a helpful part of the program.
- Aim for 7 to 14 tbsp (100 to 200 ml) of olive oil intake per week. It should replace many of the fats in your old diet.

I went into a McDonald's yesterday and said, "I'd like some fries." The girl at the counter said, "Would you like some fries with that?"

— Jay Leno

8

Recipes For The Ketogenic Mediterranean Diet

This chapter provides seven days of meals consistent with the Ketogenic Mediterranean Diet (KMD). (If you've chosen to follow the Advanced Mediterranean Diet instead, skip this chapter.) Even if you follow the guidelines and restrictions "to a T," the Ketogenic Mediterranean Diet provides lots of variety, limited mostly by your imagination. You're going to eat lots of natural, whole foods made by God, and few processed, man-made foods.

You don't even have to do any cooking if you don't want. Avoid cooking altogether by using canned fish and meats along with raw whole foods and commercially prepared nuts, cheese, olive oil, wine, and spices. But many will appreciate the added variety and tastes that cooking brings to the table.

AS SIMPLE AS YOU LIKE

When I was following the KMD myself, a typical day started with a breakfast of cooked eggs with or without bacon, sausage, pre-cooked microwaved bratwurst, or left-over steak or chicken. Lunch was a large salad tossed with both olive oil vinaigrette and canned tuna (or the salad/vinaigrette and a separate tin of sardines or kippered herring). If vinaigrette wasn't at hand, I'd just pour olive oil, vinegar, salt, and pepper into the bowl of salad, then toss. Dinner was another large salad and steak or sautéed chicken and a glass of wine. I ate my daily ounce of nuts whenever I felt like it, and I often had a couple ounces of mozzarella string cheese. If I took my lunch to work, it could be as simple as a can of tuna (eaten with some tartar sauce), an ounce of nuts, and a couple ounces of cheese. Pretty simple if you ask me.

VINAIGRETTES

A homemade vinaigrette is an easy way to get your 2–3 tbsp (30–45 ml) of olive oil daily. The basic recipe is three parts olive oil to one part vinegar. Add salt, pepper, and other spices at your whim. Blend with a whisk, or put all ingredients in a jar with a lid and shake it. Favor red wine or white wine vinegar over balsamic. Balsamic has the highest carb content of the vinegars. I suppose you could use apple cider vinegar, too. See the Special Recipes section of this chapter for a couple fancy vinaigrettes. Mix a batch and keep it in the refrigerator—it should be good for a week. You may be able to find a commercially prepared vinaigrette in the salad dressing section of the supermarket. If so, be sure the oil is predominantly olive oil (not very common) and that a serving (usually 2 tbsp) has no more than 2 g of carb. Vinaigrettes can be used on salads, drizzled on cooked or fresh vegetables, and as marinades for fish, chicken, or beef.

If you're willing to do only minimal cooking, learn how to fry and scramble eggs. For extra credit, learn how to fry or grill steak or chicken, and sauté chicken and vegetables in olive oil.

TIME-SAVING CONVENIENCE

Canned meats and fish are times-savers and often less expensive than fresh, raw products. (Worried about mercury poisoning from fish? I've been practicing medicine for over two decades and haven't seen a case of it yet.) Canned sardines are available with sauces such as tomato, jalapeno, or mustard—just be sure it doesn't add more than a couple carb grams per 4-ounce (113 g) serving. Also watch out for added carbs in canned meats (chicken, for example). Man-made processed meats (sausages, Spam, bacon, or ham, for example) may have unacceptably high added carbs: if it has over 2–3 g of carbs per 3 or 4-ounce (85–113 g) serving, take a pass and stick with natural meats.

Canned vegetables are usually OK, too. Consider canned green beans, asparagus, and spinach, for example. These are often criticized for their salt content, but the KMD is naturally low in salt and tends to lower blood pressure, so you don't have to worry about the salt in canned vegetables. Frozen vegetables are also conveniently boiled-in-the-bag or microwaved. (Oh, no . . . that's not cooking, is it?)

Finally, in 2012, the food manufacturers are responding to consumer requests for truly "natural" foods with less man-made ingredients such as high fructose corn syrup (HFCS; pure carbohydrate). Search the shelves of your supermarket and you'll find ketchup and picante sauce without HFCS.

A WEEK OF MENUS

Here are some meal ideas to get you started. Each day's menu conforms fairly well to the Ketogenic Mediterranean Diet. Digestible carb totals for each day are in the 20 to 30 gram range. Average daily calorie count is 1,850, with a range of 1,550 to 1,950. This is more than some will want or need. Just eat until you're full, not stuffed, and save the leftovers for another day. Of the total calories, average daily contribution from carbohydrate is 8%, from fat is 65%, from protein is 22%, and from alcohol is 5%. Calorie contributions from fat and protein vary quite a bit more day-to-day than do calories from carbohydrate.

Regarding olive oil, I tend to prefer extra virgin olive oil over the others. My salt choice is often potassium chloride rather than sodium chloride (table salt), which may help prevent muscle cramps sometimes seen at the start of very-low-carb eating.

"Dinner" is the evening meal, by the way.

Day 1

Breakfast: Eggs and Bratwurst

3 large eggs
1.5 tbsp (22 ml) olive oil

salt and pepper
1 (66g) pre-cooked bratwurst

Sauté eggs in the olive oil. Salt and pepper to taste. Microwave a pre-cooked bratwurst. Digestible carb grams: 2.

Lunch: Tossed Tuna Salad and Almonds

3.5 oz (100 g) lettuce
1.5 oz (42 g) chopped onion
5.5 oz (150 g) chunked tomatoes
5-oz can (140 g) of solid white albacore tuna packed
    in water (drain and discard the fluid)
1.5 tbsp (22 ml) extra virgin olive oil
½ tbsp (7.5 ml) balsamic vinegar
salt and pepper
1 oz (28 g) almonds

In a 3-qt (3 liter) bowl, put lettuce, onion, chunked tomatoes, and tuna (3.25 oz or 90 g at this point). Add the olive oil, balsamic vinegar, and salt and pepper to taste. Mix well with a fork. Enjoy almonds separately, before, during, or after salad. Digestible carb grams: 12.

Dinner: Steak and Mushrooms

1.5 tbsp (21 g or 22 ml) butter
2 tsp (10 ml) olive oil
6 oz (170 g) steak
5 oz (140 g) sliced white mushrooms
2 tsp (10 ml) Worcestershire sauce or A.1. Steak
    Sauce
5 oz (150 ml) red wine
salt and pepper

Grill or sauté (with olive oil or butter) the steak. Melt 1.5 tbsp (22 ml) of butter in pan, add mushrooms and cook over medium heat about 3 minutes, stirring frequently. Season steak and mushrooms with salt and pepper to taste. Enjoy steak with your favorite steak sauce or Worcestershire sauce, but no more than 2 g of carbs in the sauce (e.g., 2 tsp (10 ml) of A.1. Sauce or Lea & Perrins Worcestershire sauce has 2 g of carb). Digestible carb grams: 10.

Day 2

Breakfast: Mexican Eggs and Avocado

3 large eggs (50 g each)
1 tbsp (14 g or 15 ml) butter
½ cup (240 ml) Pico de Gallo a la Rosa (See Special
    Recipes at end of this chapter)
1 California avocado (135 g), peeled, seeded, and
    sliced
salt and pepper

Sauté eggs in butter. Top with ½ cup Pico de Gallo a la Rosa (see Special Recipes). May substitute for Pico de Gallo: any serving of commercial picante sauce with no more than 3 g of digestible carb (digestible carb grams = total carb grams in serving minus fiber grams in serving). Salt and pepper to taste. Digestible carb grams: 7.

Lunch: Tuna Salad Over Lettuce, with Walnuts

1 large egg (50 g)
3 oz (85 g) romaine lettuce
5-oz can of white albacore tuna packed in water
    (drain and discard the fluid)

½ oz (14 g) onion, diced (about 2 tbsp)
8-inch stalk (40 g or 20-cm stalk) of celery, diced
2 tbsp (30 ml) Miracle Whip Dressing or regular
    mayonnaise
salt and pepper
dash of lemon (optional)
1 oz (28 g) walnuts

Hard-boil a large egg, then peel and dice. Drain liquid off a 5-ounce can of white albacore tuna (net 3.5 oz or 100 g of fish); empty tuna into bowl. Add diced egg, diced onion, diced celery, and Miracle Whip Dressing or regular mayonnaise. Mix all together, with salt and pepper and/or a dash of lemon to taste. Place on bed of romaine lettuce. Enjoy walnuts around mealtime. Digestible carb grams: 9.

Dinner: Baked Trout with Snow Peas (sugar snap peas)

7 tbsp (100 g) extra virgin olive oil
5 garlic cloves (15 g), diced
1.5 tbsp (6 g) raw parsley, chopped
1 tsp (5 ml) salt
1 tsp (5 ml) black pepper
¾ fl oz (22 g or ml) lemon juice
4 leaves (1.5 g) fresh basil, chopped
16 oz (450 g) fresh trout
6 oz (170 g) snow peas (sugar snap peas)
5 oz (150 ml) white wine

This recipe provides *two* large servings of fish and *two* servings of snow peas.

In a glass or plastic bowl, mix 5 tbsp (70 g) of the extra virgin olive oil, 3 of the diced garlic cloves (9 g), the chopped raw parsley, salt, black pepper, the lemon juice, and the chopped basil. This is your marinade.

Place fresh trout filets in a medium sized (8–9" or 20–23 cm diameter) glass baking dish, then cover with marinade. Let sit in refrigerator for 1–2 hours, turning occasionally. Preheat oven to 375°F (190°C). Pull fish dish out of refrigerator once you start the preheat process. Cover glass dish with aluminum foil, then bake in oven for 20–40 minutes. Cooking time depends on your oven and the thickness of the fish. Thin filets about 1/2" (1.25 cm) thick may be done in 20–25 minutes. Thicker fish (1" or 2.5 cm)) may take 30–45 minutes. This is a judgment call. When done, it should flake apart readily with a fork. This works well for trout, salmon, cod, tilapia, and perhaps others. Consider squeezing fresh lemon juice on cooked fish for extra zing.

Now for the snow peas. Snap off and discard both tips of the snow pea pods. Sauté 2 diced garlic cloves (6 g) in olive oil over medium heat until soft, perhaps a couple minutes. To the pan add the snow peas. Salt and pepper to taste. Stir snow peas often, if not continuously, while cooking over medium heat, about 3 minutes. Enjoy 5 oz (150 ml) white wine with your meal. Digestible carb grams in wine and half the fish, half the snow peas: 11.

Day 3

Breakfast: Bacon and Eggs

3 large eggs (50 g each)
1.5 tbsp (22 ml) olive oil
6 slices pork bacon, cured (about 50 g cooked)

Fry the eggs in olive oil. Bake or fry the bacon. Digestible carb grams: 2.

Lunch: Chicken Salad Over Mixed Greens

1 large egg (50 g)
4 oz (110 g) cooked, diced chicken (canned or
    freshly sautéed in olive oil)
½ oz (14 g) raw onion, diced (about 2 tbsp)
8-inch stalk (40 g or 20-cm stalk) of raw celery,
    diced
2.5 tbsp (40 ml) Miracle Whip Dressing or regular
    Mayonnaise
2 oz (60 g) romaine lettuce
2 oz (60 g) raw baby spinach
1 oz (28 g) almonds
salt and pepper

Hard-boil an egg, then peel and dice. In a bowl,
place the chicken and add the egg, onion, celery,
and Miracle Whip Dressing or regular mayonnaise.
Mix all together, with salt and pepper and/or a dash
of lemon juice to taste. Place on bed of lettuce and
baby spinach. Enjoy almonds around mealtime or
later as a snack. Digestible carb grams: 10.

Dinner: Baked Balsamic Salmon and Green Beans

16 oz (450 g) salmon filets
salt and pepper
4 cloves (12 g) garlic, minced
1 tbsp (15 ml) olive oil
1.5 oz (45 ml) white wine for the glaze
4.5 tsp (22 ml) mustard
4 tbsp (60 ml) balsamic vinegar
1 tbsp (15 ml) granulated Splenda (or 1 packet (1g)
    of tabletop Splenda)
1.5 tbsp (22 ml) fresh chopped oregano (or 1 tsp
    (5 ml) dried oregano)
200 g canned green beans (or fresh green beans
    sautéed in olive oil/garlic)

5 oz (150 ml) dry white wine

This makes two large servings.

Preheat oven to 400°F (200°C). Line a baking sheet or pan (8" or 20 cm) with aluminum foil. Lightly salt and pepper the fish in the lined pan, with the skin side down.

Now the glaze. Sauté the minced garlic in olive oil in a small saucepan over medium heat for about three minutes, until it's soft. Then add and mix white wine (1.5 oz), mustard, vinegar, granulated Splenda, and 1/8 tsp (0.625 ml) salt. Simmer uncovered over low or medium heat until slightly thickened, about three minutes. Remove glaze from heat and spoon about half of it into a separate container for later use.

Drizzle and brush the salmon in the pan with the glaze left in the saucepan. Sprinkle the oregano on top.

Bake the fish in the oven for about 10–13 minutes, or until it flakes easily with a fork. Cooking time depends on your oven and thickness of the fish. Over-cooking the fish will toughen it and dry it out. When done, use a turner to transfer the fish to plates, leaving the skin on the foil if able. Drizzle the glaze from the separate container over the filets with a spoon, or brush it on. Don't use the unwashed brush you used earlier on the raw fish.

Heat canned green beans (200 g) on stovetop or serve at room temperature straight out of the can.

Enjoy a 5-oz glass of dry white wine with your meal. This recipe makes two servings of fish and green beans. Digestible carb grams in wine, half the fish, half the green beans: 14.

[The *balsamic* vinegar adds six g of carb to each serving. To reduce vinegar carbs to zero, you could try this recipe with red wine vinegar, white wine vinegar, or cider vinegar. I've not tried that. Digestible carbs per serving would drop to 8 g.]

Day 4

Breakfast: Steak and Avocado

4 oz (110 g) raw steak
1 California avocado, peeled, seeded, and sliced
    (136 g)
½ tbsp (7 ml) olive oil (optional)
salt and pepper
1 tbsp (15 ml) vinaigrette (see Special Recipes) or
    commercial Italian dressing (regular, not low-fat,
    with less than 2 g of carb per tbsp or 15 ml)

Cook the steak over medium heat, adding half a tbsp (7 ml) olive oil at the start if desired. Salt and pepper to taste. Peel and slice a California avocado. Dress avocado with homemade vinaigrette (see Special Recipes) or commercial Italian dressing. Salt and pepper to taste. Digestible carb grams: 4.

Lunch: Avocado Cucumber Salad

5 oz (140 g) cucumber, peeled and sliced into
    rounds
1 California avocado, peeled, seeded, and sliced
    (136 g)
2 tbsp (30 ml) AMD vinaigrette (see Special Recipes)
    or commercial Italian dressing described below

salt and pepper
dash of lime or lemon juice (optional)
1 oz walnuts

Mix the cucumber and avocado in a bowl with the AMD vinaigrette or commercial Italian dressing (regular, not low-fat, with 3 g or fewer carbs per 2 tbsp or 30 ml). Salt and pepper to taste. For extra zing, add a dash of lemon or lime juice. Enjoy the walnuts on the side now, or mid-afternoon as a snack. Digestible carb grams: 10.

Dinner: Bacon Shrimp Salad

2 slices (15 g) pork bacon, cured, cooked (or
    substitute 2 tbsp (30 ml) commercial real bacon
    bits)
2 tbsp (30 ml) AMD vinaigrette (see Special Recipes)
    or commercial Italian dressing as below
½ packet of tabletop Splenda
4 oz (110 g) fresh baby spinach
4 oz (110 g) cooked shrimp [Consider commercial
    pre-cooked, peeled shrimp to save time.]
6 oz (180 ml) dry white wine

Cook two bacon slices over medium heat, then crumble or cut in to tiny pieces (or substitute commercial real bacon bits). Add a half packet of Splenda to the AMD vinaigrette or commercial Italian dressing (regular, not low-fat, with 3 g or fewer carbs per 2 tbsp or 30 ml), then mix. On a bed of fresh baby spinach, place the cooked shrimp, then top with bacon pieces and vinaigrette. Enjoy with 6 oz dry white wine. Digestible carb grams: 9.

Day 5

Breakfast: Mexican Scrambled Eggs

4 large eggs (50 g each)
1.5 tbsp (22 ml) olive oil
4 tbsp (60 ml) Pico de Gallo a la Rosa (see Special
    Recipes) or commercial picante sauce (having 2 g
    or fewer carbs per 2 tbsp)
salt and pepper

Whisk the eggs until smooth, add salt and pepper to taste; set aside. Heat the olive oil in a medium-sized frying pan then add the eggs and cook until done, scrambling now and then. Transfer to plate and top with 4 tbsp (60 ml) Pico de Gallo a la Rosa. Digestible carb grams: 6.

Lunch: Low-Carb Chili

1 cup (240 ml) Low-Carb Chili (see Special Recipes)
1 oz (28 g) almonds

Enjoy 1 oz of almonds around mealtime or later as a snack. Digestible carb grams: 13.

Dinner: Shark and Broccoli

4 oz (110 g) shark, raw
2 cloves (3 g) garlic, peeled and diced
3 tbsp (45 ml) olive oil
1.5 cups (150 g) chopped raw broccoli
salt and pepper
6 oz (180 ml) dry white wine

Lightly salt and pepper the shark, then set aside. Sauté the garlic in 2 tbsp (30 cc) of olive oil a few minutes over medium heat. Add broccoli and sauté to your preference, adding salt and pepper to taste. Remove to a dish. Add another 1 tbsp (15 ml) olive oil to the pan and sauté the shark at medium heat until done, careful not to overcook. Enjoy with dry white wine. Digestible carb grams: 11.

Day 6

Breakfast: Chicken Salad Over Greens

1 large egg (50 g)
5-oz can (150 g) of cooked chicken (drain and
    discard liquid)
½ oz (14 g) onion (2 tbsp or 30 ml), diced
½ stick (40 g) of celery, diced
2 tbsp (30 ml) Miracle Whip Salad Dressing or
    Regular mayonnaise (not low-fat)
salt and pepper
2 oz (60 g) romaine lettuce
2 oz (60 g) raw baby spinach
dash of lemon or lime juice (optional)
1 oz (28 g) walnuts

Hard-boil the large egg, then peel and dice. Place the chicken into a bowl then add egg, diced onion, diced celery, and the Miracle Whip Salad Dressing. Mix all together, with salt and pepper and/or a dash of lemon or lime juice to taste. Place on bed of romaine lettuce and fresh baby spinach. Enjoy walnuts around mealtime or later as a snack. Digestible carb grams: 11.

Lunch: Kippered Herring and Cheese

3.5 oz (100 g) canned kippered herring
3 oz (80 g) cheese

Digestible carb grams: 2.

Dinner: Hamburger and Salad

8 oz (225 g) raw hamburger meat
1 oz (28 g) onion, finely chopped
1 tbsp (15 ml) A.1. Steak Sauce or Worcestershire
    sauce
salt and pepper
3 oz (85 g) lettuce
3 oz (85 g) tomato, cut into chunks
2 oz (60 g) cucumber, peeled and sliced
1.5 tbsp (22 ml) olive oil
½ tbsp (7 ml) vinegar

To the raw hamburger meat, add the chopped onion, A.1. Steak Sauce or Worcestershire sauce, and salt and pepper to taste. Blend thoroughly with your hands. (No particular need for *lean* hamburger; it's your choice.) Cook in pan over medium heat. While cooking, prepare your salad.

In a bowl, place the lettuce, tomato chunks, sliced cucumber, and finally, the olive oil and vinegar. Mix salad thoroughly. Salt and pepper to taste.

Enjoy with 6 oz of red wine. Digestible carb grams: 13.

Day 7

Breakfast: Brats and Tomatoes

6 oz (170 g) tomato, sliced
2 tbsp (30 ml) AMD vinaigrette (see Special Recipes)
  or commercial Italian dressing (regular, not
  low-fat, with 3 g or fewer carbs per 2 tbsp or
  30 ml)
salt and pepper
2 pre-cooked bratwursts (about 2.3 oz or 65 g each)
6 tsp (30 ml) mustard (optional)

Dress the tomato slices with the vinaigrette, plus salt and pepper to taste. Heat 2 pre-cooked bratwursts as instructed on package. Use mustard on the brats if desired. Digestible carb grams: 8.

Lunch: Easy Tuna Plus Pecans

5-oz can (140 g) of albacore tuna
2 tbsp (30 ml) Miracle Whip Salad Dressing (or real,
  high-fat mayonnaise)
1 tsp (5 ml) lemon or lime juice
1 oz (28 g) pecan halves

Drain the liquid from tuna then place tuna in a bowl. Add Miracle Whip Salad Dressing and lemon or lime juice. Mix thoroughly and enjoy. Eat 1 oz of pecan halves around mealtime or later as a snack. If you want to simplify this, forget the Miracle Whip and lemon; just use 1 oz (28 g) of commercial tartar sauce that derives at least 80% of calories from fat and has less than 3 g of carb per 2 tbsp or 30 ml. Digestible carb grams: 5.

Dinner: Ham Salad

2 oz (60 g) cooked ham, cut in to small cubes
1 oz (28 g) celery, sliced and diced
1 oz (28 g) seedless grapes (about 4 grapes), cut into
small chunks
1 oz (28 g) walnuts, coarsely crumbled
4 oz (110 g) romaine lettuce
3 tbsp AMD vinaigrette or commercial Italian,
    French, or ranch dressing having 2 or fewer
    grams of carb per 2 tbsp or 30 ml)

Lay out a bed of lettuce then sprinkle these on top:
ham, celery, grapes, and walnuts. Finish construction with AMD vinaigrette or commercial dressing.
You're done. Alternatively, substitute cooked chick-
en or steak for ham. With chicken, apple may work
better than grapes. If having a glass of wine (6 fl oz
or 180 ml) with meal, delete the grapes or the carb
count will be too high. Digestible carb grams: 10.

(When commercial dressing is used, the digestible
carb count is closer to 13 than 10 g.)

SPECIAL RECIPES

Nutrient analysis of these recipes is compliments of
SELF-NutritionData. You can analyze your own rec-
ipes there, finding the amounts of 40+ nutrients.
The web address is http://nutritiondata.self.com/.

ARIZONA'S BAKED CHEESECAKE

My daughter, Arizona, enjoys baking. I'm nudging
her into low-carb baking since I miss my sweets.

Arizona usually prepares the commercial cheese-
cakes based on a pre-mixed box: you add some

fresh ingredients, mix, then refrigerate. The baked cheesecake here is more work, but I think well worth the effort. We had fun making this together.

Ingredients for crust:

1.5 cups (226 g) ground nuts (pecan, walnut, or almond)
5.5 tbsp (82 ml) melted butter
½ tsp (2 g) ground cinnamon
1 egg white (33 g)
1 tbsp (15 ml) Granulated Splenda No Calorie Sweetener (optional)

Ingredients for filling:

24 oz (675 g) cream cheese
1 cup (230 g) sour cream
4 large eggs (50 g each)
1 cup (28 g) Granulated Splenda No Calorie Sweetener
juice from one lemon (47 g or ml)
2 tsp (10 ml) vanilla extract

Preparation

Have the following ingredients at room temperature before you start: eggs, cream cheese, and sour cream.

Preheat oven to 350°F (175°C).

First, the crust. Put ground pecans, 4 tbsp (60 ml) of the melted butter (fine to microwave briefly), cinnamon, granulated Splenda, and egg white in bowl, then blend all. Spread onto bottom of greased (with melted butter, the last 1.5 tbsp or 22 ml) 9″ (20–25 cm) springform pan. Cover with plastic wrap to aid spreading evenly; remove and discard plastic wrap after spreading the crust. Bake in 350°F (175°C) oven for 10–15 minutes then remove. Then reduce heat to 325°F (160°C).

Filling: Use a mixer on low to medium setting to beat the cream cheese until fluffy. Blend in the Splenda a little at a time, beating until creamy. Then mix in the lemon juice and vanilla extract. Gently mix in one egg at a time and beat on low speed after each egg. Mix in the sour cream last. Pour cream cheese mixture into the crusted spring-form pan. Place on the top rack in the 325°F (160°C) preheated oven for 50–60 minutes. On the rack below that, place a pie pan full of water. [The water pan and gentle handling of the eggs help prevent cracking of the final product.] When time is up, turn off the oven and open the oven door but leave the cake in the oven to cool slowly. After an hour, remove from oven. After it cools to room temperature, put it in the refrigerator to age for 24 hours.

Notes:

■ The filling has one cup of Splenda, which I estimate is one ounce (28 g). This has 96 calories, which I assume is mostly from maltodextrin rather than sucralose.
■ Many cooks just use a glass pie pan instead of the springform pan. The volume of this recipe is likely too much for a 9″ (23 cm) pie pan, so you could reduce the amounts; or make a larger pie or two smaller ones.
■ Some cooks don't bother to bake the crust first.
■ Reduce the carb count even further by omitting the crust.
■ For higher fiber, substitute flax meal for about a third or ½ of the ground nuts.

■ The Splenda in this recipe is not the same formulation as Splenda in individual serving packets.

Nutrient analysis:

Recipe makes 12 servings. Each serving has 444 calories, 8 g carbohydrate, 2 g fiber, 6 g digestible carbohydrate, 8 g protein, 43 g fat. 6% of calories are from carbohydrate, 8% from protein, 86% from fat.

LOW-CARB CHILI

It's spicy, but not hot spicy.

Ingredients

20 oz (567 g) raw ground beef, 80% lean meat/20% fat
20 oz (567 g) raw pork Italian sausage
1 large onion
14.5 oz (411 g) canned diced tomatoes
4 oz (113 g) tomato paste
1 tbsp (15 ml) dry unsweetened cocoa powder
5 garlic cloves
½ tsp (2.5 ml) salt
¼ tsp (1.2 ml) ground allspice
2 tbsp (30 ml) chili powder
¼ tsp (1.2 ml) ground cinnamon
½ tbsp (7.5 ml) ground cumin
¼ tsp (1.2 ml) ground cayenne pepper
2 packets (1 g per packet) Splenda tabletop sweetener
1 cup (240 ml) water

Preparation

Cut the Italian sausage into small pieces. Sauté the sausage, ground beef, onions, and garlic in a large pot. Don't just brown the meat, cook it thoroughly. When done, drain off the fat if desired. Add the remainder of ingredients, bring to a boil, then simmer for about an hour. Add additional water if the chili looks too thick. Makes eight cups. Serving size is one cup (240 ml).

Nutrient Analysis:

Recipe makes 8 servings of 1 cup (240 ml). Each serving has 492 calories, 14 g carbohydrate, 3 g fiber, 11 g digestible carbohydrate, 24 g protein, 38 g fat. 10% of calories are from carbohydrate, 21% from protein, 69% from fat.

Notes: Analysis is based on fat not being drained from the cooked meat. Calorie count and calories from fat would be a bit lower if you drained off fat. Peeled and sliced cold cucumbers make a nice side dish. If your children or housemates aren't eating low-carb, they may enjoy the chili mixed 50:50 with cheese macaroni, and buttered cornbread on the side.

PICO DE GALLO A LA ROSA

Try this, for example, over fried eggs.

Ingredients

6 oz (170 g) tomatoes
2 oz (56 g) onion
1 jalapeno pepper (14 g)
3–4 tbsp (2 g) cilantro
salt

Preparation

Chop all vegetables very finely. Use the entire jala-peno, including seeds, but not the stem. If you pre-fer less spicy heat, use less jalapeno and discard the seeds. Combine all ingredients after chopping. Salt to taste. Eat at room temperature, chilled, or heated at medium heat in a saucepan (about 5 minutes, until jalapenos lose their intense green color). Makes 1.25 cups.

Nutrient Analysis:

Recipe makes about three servings of ½ cup (120 ml) each. One serving has 80 calories, 4 g carb, 1 g fiber, 3 g digestible carb, 1 g protein, minimal fat. 83% of calories are from carbohydrate, 10% from protein, 7% from fat.

ALMOND POUND CAKE

My son, Paul, and I had a great time making this when he was 11-years-old, around the time he an-nounced he "might be interested in a career as a culinary professional." This cake was our first joint baking project.

2 cups (224 g) almond flour
½ cup (113 g) butter at room temperature
4 oz (116 g) cream cheese at room temperature
1 cup (28 g) Splenda Granulated No Calorie Swee-
    tener
6 eggs, medium size (44 g each), at room tempera-
    ture
1 tsp (5 ml) baking powder
1 tbsp (15 ml) lemon zest (or 1.5 tsp or 7 ml lemon
    extract)
1 tsp (5 ml) vanilla extract

If you can't find almond flour, make your own by grinding almonds into the consistency of a flour. You can do this in a blender or electric coffee bean grinder.

Preparation

Preheat oven to 350°F (175°C).

Mix the butter, cream cheese, and Splenda with a hand-held or table-top mixer, then beat in the eggs one at a time, mixing thoroughly after each egg. In a separate container, mix the baking powder into the almond flour. Add the almond flour a little at a time into the butter/sour cream bowl, beating as you go. Then mix in vanilla extract and lemon zest. Pour into a 9-inch (22-24 cm) cake pan greased with butter, vegetable oil, or Baker's Joy Baking Spray, then bake at 350°F (175°C). for 35-40 minutes.

Nutrient Analysis:

Recipe makes 12 servings. Each serving has 248 calories, 5 g carbohydrate, 1 g fiber, 4 g digestible carbohydrate, 5 g protein, 18 g fat. 27% of calories are from carbohydrate, 9% from protein, 64% from fat.

AMD VINAIGRETTE

Try this on salads, fresh vegetables, or as a marinade for chicken, fish, or beef. If using as a marinade, keep the entree/marinade combo in the refrigerator for 4–24 hours. Seasoned vinaigrettes taste even better if you let them sit for several hours after preparation.

Ingredients

1 clove (3 g) garlic
juice from ½ lemon (23 g or ml)
a third of a cup (78 ml) olive oil
2 tbsp (8 g) fresh parsley
½ tsp (2.5 ml)) salt
½ tsp (2.5 ml) yellow mustard
½ tsp (1.2 ml) paprika
2 tbsp (30 ml) vinegar, red wine,

Preparation

In a bowl, combine all ingredients and whisk together. Alternatively, you can put all ingredients in
a jar with a lid and shake vigorously. Let sit at room
temperature for an hour, for flavors to meld. Then
refrigerate. It should "keep" for at least 5 days in
refrigerator. Shake before using. Servings per batch:
3.

Nutrient Analysis:

Recipe makes 3 servings (2 tbsp or 30 ml per serving). Each serving has 220 calories, 2 g digestible
carb, almost no fiber, negligible protein, 24 g fat. 3%
of calories are from carbohydrate, 97% from fat.

MUSTARD VINAIGRETTE

Try this on salads, fresh vegetables, or as a marinade for chicken, fish, or beef. If using as a marinade, keep the entree/marinade combo in the refrigerator for 4–24 hours.

Ingredients

3 tsp (15 ml) yellow mustard, yellow

¾ cup (177 ml) olive oil
½ tsp (2.5 ml) salt
½ tsp (2.5 ml) pepper (fresh ground if available)
¼ cup (60 ml) cider vinegar

Preparation

Mix all ingredients in a jar with a lid. Shake vigorously to create an emulsion. Let sit at room temperature for an hour, for flavors to meld. Then refrigerate. Should "keep" for at least 5 days in refrigerator. Shake before using. Makes one cup.

Nutrient Analysis:

Recipe makes one cup (8 servings of 2 tbsp each). Each serving has 182 calories, negligible carbs, zero protein, 20 g fat. 1% of calories are from carbohydrate, 99% from fat.

You'll find sources of free online low-carb recipes back in chapter six.

There are no secrets to success. It is the result of preparation, hard work, learning from failure.
— General Colin Powell

9

Recipes For The Advanced Mediterranean Diet

(If you chose to try the Ketogenic Mediterranean Diet rather than the Advanced Mediterranean Diet, see chapters five and eight instead.)

The nutrient composition of the Advanced Mediterranean Diet approximates that of the Mediterranean region in the mid-20th century. This doesn't mean you must eat specific dishes associated with the Mediterranean, such as tabbouleh, couscous, spaghetti, ravioli, shish kabob, and hummus. You may, but it's not required in order to reap the health benefits of Mediterranean-style eating. Your new diet will be characterized by whole grains, fruits, vegetables, legumes, nuts, olive oil and other beneficial fats, fish, optional wine, and relatively small amounts of meat, poultry, and dairy products. When you have a choice, choose natural, fresh, whole, minimally processed items.

You don't have to cook anything to follow the Advanced Mediterranean Diet. Now, I'm not suggesting you eat raw eggs, meat, chicken or anything else that requires cooking for safety or to enhance palatability. You could choose, for example, canned tuna or meat substitutes such as nuts or canned beans, and avoid cooking altogether.

Odds are, however, you're already cooking at least a little, such as heating canned or frozen vegetables on a stove or in a microwave oven. Your meal options certainly increase if you're willing to cook.

A typical day's intake could start with Old Fashioned Quaker Oats that you cook for five minutes, then add fresh or canned fruit (300 calories total). For lunch: 2 ounces of nuts plus an apple and a banana (560 calories). For dinner: fresh broccoli sautéed in olive oil spiced with garlic, chicken breast sautéed in olive oil and garlic, and whole grain bread with Smart Balance Buttery Spread (960 calories). This is quick, simple cuisine. Make it as fancy as you wish within the guidelines provided in chapter seven.

You'll notice that many of these recipes utilize low-fat versions of dairy products or meat. That's to cut back a bit on calories while making room for more fiber and plant-based nutrients. This won't be necessary when you get down to your goal weight.

You don't count calories; you check off boxes on your Daily Log as you eat. For the recipes that follow, I tell you which boxes to mark since it's not always obvious. See "Box breakdown" at the end of each recipe. Sometimes you mark just half a box. Fill in the other half when you eat later.

Your choice of foods on the Advanced Mediterranean Diet is based on Table 5.1, Food Choices & Serving Sizes, in chapter seven. Note the great variety. This isn't a high-protein diet, high-fat diet, low-fat diet, low-carbohydrate diet, or take-this-pill-and-eat-anything-you-want diet.

BREAKFAST RECIPES

Cereal & Fruit

Boxed cereal: ¼ cup (60 ml) Post Grape Nuts or 1 cup (240 ml) Cheerios or ½ cup (120 ml) raisin bran or 1 oz (30 g) shredded wheat cereal or 100 calorie serving of any whole grain breakfast cereal containing at least 3 grams of fiber), plus 1 cup (240 ml) low-fat milk, plus 1 banana.

Box breakdown: 1 grain, 1 milk, 1 fruit (290 cal)

Oat Porridge

Bring 1½ cups (360 ml) water to a boil, add ¾ cup (180 ml) Old Fashioned Quaker Oats and a pinch of salt. Simmer about five minutes over low or medium heat, stirring now and then. Remove from heat and add a fruit serving: chopped or grated medium apple, banana, or peach, ½ cup (120 ml) unsweetened applesauce, 1/8 cup (30 ml) raisins, or 1 cup (240 ml) strawberries, blackberries, or blueberries.

Box breakdown: 2 grains, 1 fruit (280 cal)

Toast & Yogurt

Toast two whole grain bread slices in toaster, then spread with 1 tbsp (15 ml) butter or Smart Balance Buttery Spread. ½ cup (120 ml) low-fat yogurt.

Box breakdown: 2 grains, 1 fat, 1 milk (420 cal)

Toast & Fruit

Toast two whole grain bread slices in toaster, then spread with 1 tbsp (15 ml) butter or Smart Balance Buttery Spread. Enjoy with an apple, banana, or orange.

Box breakdown: 2 grains, 1 fruit, 1 fat (390 cal)

Crunchy Yogurt

Add ¼ cup (60 ml) Post Grape Nuts to 1 cup (240 ml) low-fat yogurt. Stir. Or add Grape Nuts gradually as you eat the yogurt.

Box breakdown: 1 grain, 2 milks (320 cal)

Nutty Yogurt

Add ½ oz (15 g) chopped nuts (pecans, walnuts, almonds) or sun-flower seeds to 1 cup (240 ml) low-fat yogurt.

Box breakdown: 1 fat, 2 milk (330 cal)

Egg Sandwich

Fry two eggs in 1 tbsp (15 ml) butter or Smart Balance Buttery Spread. Toast two slices whole grain bread in toaster then spread one piece with 2 tbsp (30 ml) Miracle Whip Dressing. Place eggs between toast slices.

Box breakdown: 2 grains, 2 fats, 1 protein (620 cal)

Scrambled Eggs & Fruit

No, the fruit doesn't go in the scrambled eggs. Crack two eggs into a bowl, add a dash of milk, salt and pepper to taste, whisk with a fork until uniform. Sauté 1–2 tbsp (15–30 ml) chopped onion and bell pepper in 1 tbsp (15 ml) butter or Smart Balance Buttery Spread. Add eggs to the sauté pan and cook over medium heat until firm, stirring occasionally. Serve with 1 cup (240 ml) cubed honeydew melon or cantaloupe.

Box breakdown: 1 fruit, 1 fat, 1 protein (390 cal)

Bacon & Eggs & Fruit

Crack two eggs into a bowl, add a dash of milk, salt and pepper to taste, whisk with a fork until uniform. Melt 1 tbsp (15 ml) butter or Smart Balance Buttery Spread in a small frying pan. Pour the eggs into the pan, add 1 level tbsp (15 ml) bacon bits, cook over medium heat until firm, stirring occasionally. Serve with a banana, apple, or orange, or 1 cup (240 ml) cubed cantaloupe or honeydew melon.

Box breakdown: 1 fruit, 2 fats, 1 protein (500 cal)

Cottage Cheese with Fruit

To 1 cup (240 ml) low-fat cottage cheese add one diced peach or apple, or 1 cup (240 ml) blueberries or blackberries, or ½ cup (120 ml) unsweetened applesauce, or other fruit serving of your choice.

Box breakdown: 1 fruit, 2 milk (300 cal)

Breakfast Burrito

1–2 tbsp (15–30 ml) green bell pepper, diced
1 tbsp (15 ml) onion, diced
1 egg
1½ tsp (7 ml) milk
salt & pepper
1 tsp (5 ml) Smart Balance Buttery Spread or
    butter
7" (18 cm) whole wheat tortilla
1 tbsp (15 ml) Pace Picante Sauce

In a 7–8 inch (20 cm) non-stick frying pan, sauté bell pepper and onion in Smart Balance or butter. Whisk egg and milk in a bowl, then add to the pan and cook like scrambled eggs over medium heat. Salt and pepper to taste. When done, transfer to a clean bowl. Use the pan to heat a tortilla. Put tortilla on a plate, load eggs and picante sauce on the tortilla, then roll it up and enjoy.

Box breakdown: 1 grain, ½ fat, ½ protein (250 cal)

Whole Wheat Fruity Pancakes

1 cup (240 ml) Krusteaz Wheat & Honey
    Complete Pancake Mix
¾ cup (180 ml) cold water
½ cup (120 ml) berries or diced fruit
    (blueberries, blackberries, raspberries, diced
    strawberries, apple, or banana)
PAM Cooking Spray or Mazola Pure Cooking
Spray
        (canola or butter flavor)
4½ tbsp (65 ml) lite syrup
2 tbsp (30 ml) Smart Balance Buttery Spread

Mix Krusteaz Pancake Mix with water in a bowl as directed on package. Blend with a wire whisk or fork. Add a little more water if batter seems too thick. Do not over-mix. Batter will be slightly lumpy. Gently blend in the fruit.

Pour a little less than ¼ cup (60 ml) batter per pancake onto a preheated griddle (medium heat, 375°F or 190°C) lightly coated with PAM or Mazola Pure. Aim for pancakes 3½ or 4" (10 cm) diameter. Cook pancakes until golden brown, roughly 1½ minutes per side, turning only once if possible. Remove from heat. Spread pancakes with a light coat of Smart Balance, ½ tsp (3 ml) per 2–3 pancakes, then pour ½ tbsp (7 ml) lite syrup over each pancake. Bon appétit! Allow leftovers to cool to room temperature, then store refrigerated in a baggie. Reheat in microwave.

Servings per batch: 2–3 (about eight pancakes, 3½–4" (10 cm) diameter)

Serving size: three pancakes with Smart Balance & syrup

Calories per pancake with Smart Balance & syrup: 95 cal

Box breakdown: 3 grains *or* 2 grains and 1 fat (280 cal)

LUNCH RECIPES

Kippered Herring Sandwich

Build this with two slices whole grain bread, mustard, and 4 oz (113 g) canned kippered herring. Alternatively, use tuna or sardines.

Box breakdown: 2 grains, 1 protein (400 cal)

Nuts & Fruit

4 oz (113 g) nuts and an apple, orange, or banana.
    Box breakdown: 2 proteins, 1 fruit (480 cal)

Tomatoes & Crackers

Slice two medium tomatoes, drizzle with 1–2 tbsp (15–30ml) salad dressing. Serve with five Triscuit Original Crackers.
    Box breakdown: 1 grains, 1 vegetable, 1 fat (270 cal)

Water Chestnut Salad

    2 cups (480 ml) lettuce
    ½ cup (120 ml) water chestnuts
    1 celery stalk, sliced
    10 ripe black olives, medium sized
    2 tbsp (30 ml) salad dressing

Mix everything in bowl. The celery and lettuce are daily bonus foods that incur no charge in terms of calories.
    Box breakdown: 2 vegetables, 1 fat (230 cal)

Cheese, Crackers, Fruit, and Yogurt

Slice 1 oz (30 g) cheese into thirds and eat with three Ry Krisp Natural Crackers. ½ cup (120 ml) low-fat yogurt and 12 raw cherries or other fruit serving.
    Box breakdown: 1 grain, 1 fruit, 1 fat, 1 milk (400 cal)

Tomato Salad

2 cups (480 ml) lettuce
1 medium tomato, sliced into chunks
1 raw carrot, sliced into chunks
1 celery stalk, sliced into chunks
2 tbsp (30 ml) salad dressing

Mix all ingredients in bowl. The lettuce and celery are "free" items with near zero calories.

Box breakdown: 1 vegetable, 1 fat (170 cal)

Mexitalian Bean Salad

1 15-oz (425 g)) can black beans, drained and
    rinsed
1 15-oz (425 g) can kidney beans, drained and
    rinsed
1 15-oz (425 g) can whole kernel yellow corn,
    drained
1 15-oz (425 g) can diced tomatoes, drained
    (or 3 tomatoes, diced, and seeded if
    desired)
1 red bell pepper, seeded and chopped
1 green bell pepper, seeded and chopped
6–8 green onions, chopped
1 cup (240 ml) fresh cilantro, chopped
¼ cup (60 ml) extra virgin olive oil
¼ cup (60 ml) red wine vinegar
1 garlic clove, minced or crushed
1 jalapeno pepper, minced
2 limes, juiced
2 tbsp (30 ml) white sugar
2 tsp (10 ml) salt
1 tsp (5 ml) ground cumin
½ tsp (3 ml) fresh ground black pepper

In a small bowl, whisk together vinegar, olive oil, lime juice, sugar, garlic, salt, black pepper, cumin and jalapeno. Set this dressing aside.

In a large bowl, combine beans, corn, onions, bell peppers, tomatoes, and cilantro.

Pour dressing over ingredients in large bowl, then mix well, but gently. Chill in refrigerator for at least two hours, ideally eight or 12 hours. Serve cold. This goes well with something crunchy, such as crackers or celery sticks.

Servings per batch: 8

Serving size: 1 cup

Box breakdown: 3 vegetables, ½ fat (245 cal)

Bread & Butter Sandwich with Fruit

Build a sandwich with 2 slices whole grain bread and 1 tbsp (15 ml) butter or Smart Balance Buttery Spread. Serve with two medium plums or other fruit serving.

Box breakdown: 2 grains, 1 fruit, 1 fat (390 cal)

Avocado Cucumber Salad

½ sliced avocado, one sliced cucumber, both drizzled with 1–2 tbsp (15–30 ml) salad dressing. Salt and pepper to taste.

Box breakdown: 2 vegetables, 1 fat (230 cal)

Toasted Peanut Butter Sandwich

2 tbsp (30 ml) peanut butter between two slices of toasted whole grain bread.

Box breakdown: 2 grains, 1 protein (400 cal)

Eggs, Crackers, and Vegetable Juice

Two hard-boiled eggs (see cookbooks by Becker, Bittman, or Crocker under "Recommended Further Reading") salted to taste, served with five Triscuit Original Crackers and 10 oz (285 g) canned vegetable juice such as V8 100% Vegetable Juice.

Box breakdown: 1 grain, 1 vegetable, 1 protein (360 cal)

Yogurt & Fruit

1 cup (240 ml) low-fat yogurt served with an orange or other fruit serving.

Box breakdown: 1 fruit, 2 milks (300 cal)

Chicken Salad on Ry

4 oz (113 g) canned chicken (packed in water)
2 tbsp (30 ml) Miracle Whip Dressing
½ celery stalk, finely chopped
1–2 tbsp (15–30 ml) onion, finely chopped
6 Ry Krisp Natural Crackers (or 10 Triscuit crackers)

Mix first four ingredients together, then spoon onto crackers.

Box breakdown: 2 grains, 1 fat, 1 protein (510 cal)

Tuna Salad on Ry

Same as above except use canned tuna.

Box breakdown: 2 grains, 1 fat, 1 protein (510 cal)

Sunny's Hummus on Bread or Crackers

1 15-oz (425 g) can of garbanzo beans, drained
1 tbsp (15 ml) olive oil
1/8 cup (30 ml) fresh lemon juice (about ½ lemon)
3 garlic cloves, minced
1 tbsp (15 ml) fresh parsley, chopped
1 tsp (5 ml) fresh basil, chopped, or ½ tsp dried basil
salt and pepper to taste
1 slice whole grain bread or 5 Triscuit Original crackers or 3 Ry Krisp Natural crackers

Combine all ingredients except bread and crackers in a blender or food processor; blend into a smooth paste consistency. Add a small amount of water if it seems too thick. Spread onto bread or crackers.
  Servings of hummus per batch: 3
  Serving size: 1/3 cup (80 ml) hummus (170 cal) plus bread or crackers (100 cal)
  Box breakdown: 1 grain, 2 veggie, ½ fat (275 cal)

AMD Vinaigrette

1/3 cup (80 ml) extra virgin olive oil
2 tbsp (30 ml) red wine vinegar
2 tbsp (30 ml) parsley, fresh, chopped
½ tsp (2 ml) salt
¼ tsp (1 ml) pepper, freshly ground
½ tsp (2 ml) Dijon mustard
¼ tsp (1 ml) paprika
juice of ½ lemon
1 garlic clove, minced

In a bowl, combine all ingredients and whisk together. Alternatively, you can put all ingredients in jar with a lid and shake vigorously. This tastes even better if you let it sit for several hours before using as a salad dressing or drizzling over fresh or cooked vegetables. Refrigerate any remaining.

Servings per batch: 6
Serving size: 1 tbsp
Box breakdown: 1 fat (110 cal)

Advanced Chicken Salad

10 oz (280 g) chunk chicken, canned in water, drained
½ mild onion, thinly sliced. Consider red or Vidalia onions, or 3 green onions
2 cups (480 ml) potatoes, new or red, cut into ½ to 1-inch (2 cm) chunks after scrubbing and rinsing
15 olives, black
8 oz or 2 cups (225 g or 480 ml) green beans, fresh, cut in 2 to 3-inch (5–7 cm) segments
1–2 tbsp (15–30 ml) capers (optional)
3 tomatoes, cut into wedges
3 celery stalks, cut into 1/3-inch (1 cm) segments
Romaine lettuce or fresh, raw spinach (optional)
2 tbsp (30 ml) parsley, fresh, chopped
½ tsp (2 ml) salt
¼ tsp (1 ml) pepper, freshly ground
1/3 cup (80 ml) extra virgin olive oil
2 tbsp (30 ml) red wine vinegar
½ tsp (2 ml) Dijon mustard
¼ tsp (1 ml) paprika
½ lemon, juiced
1 garlic clove, minced

Prepare vinaigrette first: in a bowl, combine garlic, salt, pepper, paprika, lemon juice, mustard, vinegar, parsley, and olive oil. Whisk together and set aside. You will use only ½ of this today. Use the remainder as a salad dressing or drizzle over fresh vegetables.

Boil potatoes in lightly salted water until cooked, about 15 minutes. You want them cooked, but still firm. Drain and set aside to cool.

Trim the ends off the green beans, cut into 2 to 3-inch (5–7 cm) segments, and place them in a pan of boiling, lightly salted water. Cook for 2–3 minutes. Drain and rinse under cold water.

In a large bowl, combine potatoes, green beans, tuna, tomato wedges, olives, capers, onion, celery, and only ½ of the vinaigrette. Add the vinaigrette last. Gently mix to coat ingredients with vinaigrette. Serve on a bed of lettuce or spinach now, or after two hours chilling in refrigerator.

Servings per batch: 4

Serving size: 1½ cups (360 ml)

Box breakdown: 1 veggie, 1 fat, ½ protein (235 cal)

Tabbouleh

1 cup (240 ml) bulgur wheat
2 cucumbers, peeled and finely chopped
3 tomatoes, finely diced
5 green onions with some of the green, finely chopped
3 garlic cloves, minced
¼ cup (60 ml) fresh mint leaves, finely chopped
2 cups (480 ml) fresh parsley, finely chopped
1/3 cup (80 ml) extra virgin olive oil
1/3 cup (80 ml) lemon juice
½ tsp (2 ml) fresh ground black pepper
¼ tsp (1 ml) nutmeg
½ tsp (2 ml) cinnamon

1 tsp (5 ml) salt
1 tsp (5 ml) white sugar

Place bulgur in a bowl then add 1 cup (240 ml) boiling water. Set this aside for 30 minutes while the bulgur soaks up the water. Prepare the cucumbers, garlic, onions, lemon juice, parsley, and mint. You will dice the tomatoes later.

In a large mixing bowl, combine the bulgur, cucumbers, onions, garlic, parsley, mint, lemon juice, olive oil, sugar, cinnamon, nutmeg, pepper, and salt. Toss the mixture until uniform, then cover and refrigerate at least six hours. Just before serving, add the tomatoes and toss again. The tomatoes get mushy if you add them earlier. Serve cold or at room temperature.

Servings per batch: 8
Serving size: ¾ cup (180 ml)
Box breakdown: ½ grain, ½ vegetable, 1 fat (185 cal)

DINNER IDEAS

Spaghetti with Sunny's Sauce

1 garlic clove, chopped
1 tbsp (15 ml) olive oil
1 tbsp (15 ml) fennel seed
¾ lb (340 g) bulk Italian sausage
½ lb (225 g) Italian sausage links, sliced into ½–1" (2 cm) segments
2 large fresh basil leaves, chopped
4 jars (1 lb, 10 oz (740 g) jars holding 3 cups or 720 ml) Chunky Ragú Mushroom & Green Pepper Sauce

In a 4 or 5-quart (4 l) pot, sauté garlic and fennel seed, stirring constantly until garlic is lightly browned. Add sausage to the pot and cook over medium heat. Add chopped basil after the meat is about half done. Drain excess fluid after meat is thoroughly cooked. Then add the Ragú to the meat in the pot. Simmer on low heat, stirring occasionally, for 2½ hours. It's not quite as tasty if you eat it after less simmering. Cook whole wheat spaghetti as per directions on box.

Sauce servings per batch: 17

Serving size: 2/3 cup (160 ml) sauce (250 cal) on 1 cup cooked spaghetti (200 cal)

Box breakdown: 2 grain, 2 veggie, 1 fat (450 cal)

Pesto Spaghetti with Brussels Sprouts on the Side

whole wheat spaghetti
Buitoni brand Pesto With Basil
Green Giant Baby Brussels Sprouts & Butter
    Sauce

Cook whole wheat spaghetti as instructed on box, then set aside. As spaghetti is cooking and when it is about half done, microwave Green Giant Baby Brussels Sprouts & Butter Sauce as on box, then serve 1 cup (240 ml). Or substitute a vegetable serving of your choice

Stir thoroughly a container of Buitoni brand Pesto With Basil (found in the refrigerated food section of most supermarkets, by the refrigerated fresh pasta, containing 300 cal per ¼ cup or 60 ml). Add 1 tbsp (15 ml) pesto to 1 cup (240 ml) of cooked spaghetti, then toss to coat spaghetti with pesto.

Save leftover plain spaghetti in the refrigerator. To re-heat later, boil water then add spaghetti and cook for 30–40 seconds. Drain spaghetti and add pesto.

Box breakdown: 2 grains, 1 vegetable, 1 fat (370 cal)

Sunny's Santa Fe Soup

1 lb (454 g) ground beef, raw, lean (85 percent lean, 15 percent fat)
½ cup (120 ml) onion, diced
1 garlic clove, diced
ground pepper
1 packet (2 oz or 60 g) Hidden Valley Original Ranch Salad Dressing and Seasoning mix
1 16-oz (454 g) can black beans
1 16-oz (454 g) can light red kidney beans
1 16-oz (454 g) can dark red kidney beans
1 28-oz (795 g) can tomatoes, diced (Hunt's)
2 packets (1.25 oz or 35 g each packet) McCormick Original Taco Seasoning Mix
1 15¼-oz (432 g) can white corn (Del Monte Fresh Cut)
1 15¼-oz (432 g) whole kernel yellow corn (Del Monte Fresh Cut)
4 oz (120 ml) water
½ tbsp (7 ml) sour cream per serving
1 sprinkle of fresh-cut chives per serving

In a 5 or 6-quart (5 l) pot, brown the crumbled ground beef (i.e., pan-fry without oil) along with the garlic, onion, and pepper to taste. When finished cooking, drain and discard the excess fluid. Add the Ranch Seasoning and Taco Seasoning, then mix well. Next add the beans, corn, and tomatoes along with all the juices in the cans. Add 4 oz (120 ml) water. Simmer for 1½ hours. Serve 1 cupful (240 ml) in a bowl with ½ tbsp (7 ml) sour cream in the center, then sprinkle with chives.

Servings per batch: 17 cups
Serving size: 1 cup (240 ml)
Box breakdown: 2 veggies, ½ protein (200 cal)
(Or count as 1 protein)

Horace's Vegetarian Chili

1½ cups (360 ml) chopped green bell pepper
1½ cups (360 ml) chopped onion
2 cloves garlic, minced
½ cup (120 ml) chopped celery
2 tbsp (30 ml) vegetable oil
1 tbsp (15 ml) chili powder (use less for milder chili)
2 tsp (10 ml) ground cumin
½ tsp (2 ml) ground red pepper
2 14.5-oz (410 g) cans diced tomatoes, undrained
2 16-oz (454 g) cans pinto beans, undrained
1 15-oz (425 g) can black beans, undrained

In a 3–4 quart (3.5 l) pot, sauté onion, bell pepper, and celery with the vegetable oil until tender. Add tomatoes, chili powder, cumin, and ground red pepper, then stir well. Blend one can of pinto beans in a blender until smooth, then add to the pot. Add remaining cans of beans to the pot, bring to a boil, reduce heat and simmer for 30 minutes.

Servings per batch: 9½
Serving size: 1 cup (240 ml)
Box breakdown: 3 veggies, or count as 1 protein (170 cal)

Pasta Primavera

1 lb (dry weight) (454 g) whole wheat pasta
4 cloves garlic, chopped
3 tbsp (45 ml) olive oil

1 cup (240 ml) carrots (sliced baby carrots or
¼" (½ cm) thick sliced adult carrots)
8 oz (225 g) sugar snap peas (slice off the very
tips)
12 oz (340 g) broccoli florets
½ cup (120 ml) sweet green (bell) peppers, sliced
or chopped
½ cup (120 ml) sweet red (bell) peppers, sliced or
chopped
garlic salt
Parmesan cheese to sprinkle
32 cherry or grape tomatoes

While heating water to cook pasta, prepare the peas, carrots, broccoli and garlic as above. Once you put the pasta in boiling water to cook, you start sautéing vegetables. The pasta will be done in 10–12 minutes. In a large frying pan, lightly sauté the garlic in 2 tbsp (30 ml) olive oil. Don't brown the garlic. Add carrots, beans, and peppers. Continue sautéing, stirring continuously for about five minutes—more or less depending on how firm you like your veggies. Add the broccoli and cook a little longer. Season to taste with garlic salt. Set these cooked vegetables aside in a large bowl.

To the empty frying pan, add 1 tbsp (15 ml) olive oil and a pinch of garlic salt. Heat briefly.

Your pasta should be about done. Drain it and add to the large bowl containing the vegetables. Add the hot olive oil and mix all together. Serve 1½ cups (360 ml) on a plate or bowl, add four cherry tomatoes, sprinkle lightly with Parmesan cheese and enjoy. Black olives go well with this dish, but you must account for the calories separately (10 cal per olive). Try the leftovers cold, as pasta salad.
   Servings per batch: 8
   Serving size: 1½ cups (360 ml)

Box breakdown: 2 grains, 1 veggie, ½ fat (300 cal)

Salad Nicoise

- 8 oz (225 g) albacore (white) tuna, canned in water, drained
- ½ mild onion, thinly sliced. Consider red or Vidalia onions, or 5 green onions
- 2 cups (480 ml) potatoes, new or red, cut into ½ to 1-inch chunks after scrubbing and rinsing
- 15 olives, black or nicoise
- 8 oz or 2 cups (225 g or 480 ml) green beans, fresh, cut in 2 to 3-inch (6 cm) segments
- 1–2 tbsp (15–30 ml) capers (optional)
- 3 tomatoes, cut into wedges
- Romaine lettuce or fresh, raw spinach (optional)
- 2 tbsp (30 ml) parsley, fresh, chopped
- ½ tsp (2 ml) salt
- ¼ tsp (1 ml) black pepper, freshly ground
- 1/3 cup (80 ml) extra virgin olive oil
- 2 tbsp (30 ml) red wine vinegar
- ½ tsp (2 ml) Dijon mustard
- ¼ tsp (1 ml) paprika
- ½ lemon, juiced
- 1 garlic clove, minced

Prepare vinaigrette first: in a bowl, combine garlic, salt, pepper, paprika, lemon juice, mustard, vinegar, parsley, and olive oil. Whisk together and set aside. You will use only ½ of this today. Use the remainder as a salad dressing or drizzle over fresh vegetables.

Boil potatoes in lightly salted water until cooked, about 15 minutes. You want them cooked, but still firm. Drain and set aside to cool.

Trim the ends off the green beans, cut into 2 to 3-inch (6 cm) segments, and place them in a pan of boiling, lightly salted water. Cook for 2–3 minutes. Drain and rinse under cold water.

In a large bowl, combine everything: potatoes, green beans, tuna, tomato wedges, olives, capers, onion, and only ½ of the vinaigrette. Add the vinaigrette last. Gently mix to coat ingredients with vinaigrette. Serve on a bed of lettuce or spinach now, or after two hours chilling in refrigerator.

This recipe omits the anchovies and hard-boiled eggs served with classic Salad Nicoise. The tuna counts as one of your twice weekly fish servings.
Servings per batch: 4
Serving size: 1½ cups (360 ml)
Box breakdown: 1 veggie, 1 fat, ½ protein (235 cal)

Moroccan Beef Stew

1½ pounds (680 g) raw lean beef, in ½ to 1-inch (2 cm) cubes (use select or choice grade of top round, top sirloin, or sirloin tip)
2 tbsp (30 ml) olive oil
4 carrots, peeled and sliced into ¼ to 1/3-inch (½ cm) thick rounds
2 red onions, chopped
3 garlic cloves, minced
1 15-oz (425 g) can diced tomatoes
1 15-oz (425 g) can chickpeas (garbanzo beans), drained and rinsed
2 cups (480 ml) beef broth (e.g., Swanson lower sodium beef broth, 100% fat free)
1 cup (240 ml) black olives, pitted and halved
2 tsp (10 ml) brown sugar

1 lemon, juice only
1½ tsp (7 ml) zest of lemon (optional)
½ cup (120 ml) cilantro, chopped
2 tsp (10 ml) ground cumin
1 tbsp (15 ml) paprika
1½ tsp (7 ml) ground cinnamon
1 tbsp (5 ml) salt
2 tsp (10 ml) ground black pepper
1½ cups (360 ml) water

Heat oil over medium-high heat in a 3- or 4-quart (3.5 l) stockpot or saucepot. Choose one with a lid to use later.

Sprinkle beef with salt and pepper, then carefully add beef to the hot oil in the pan. Keeping the heat on medium-high, brown the meat on all sides, which will take five to eight minutes. Remove meat and set aside.

To the brown juice remaining in the pan, add garlic and onion. Cook over medium-high heat until onions are soft.

Add back to the pan the cooked meat along with tomatoes, water, broth, carrots, chickpeas, spices, sugar, lemon zest, and olives. Bring to a boil then reduce to a simmer and cook covered for an hour, stirring occasionally. Cook for an additional 30–60 minutes if meat is still tough. Add more water while cooking if stew is too thick. Add cilantro and lemon juice just before serving.

Servings per batch: 10
Serving size: 1 cup (240 ml)
Box breakdown: 2½ veggies, ½ protein (255 cal)

Pasta e Fagioli

4 tbsp (60ml) olive oil
4 garlic cloves, minced
1½ cup (360 ml) chopped celery (about 3 stalks)
1 cup (240 ml) chopped red onion
3 carrots, large, julienned, 1½ inch-long (4 cm)
    strips
12 oz (340 g) bulk sweet Italian sausage (or use
    link Italian sausage after removal of the
    casing). Italian sausage is fatty: 60–75
    percent of calories are from fat. Buy as lean
    as you can.
3 15-oz (425 g) cans diced tomatoes, undrained
1 15-oz (425 g) can cannellini beans, drained
    and rinsed (alternatively, use white, navy, or
    great northern beans)
1 15-oz (425 g) can red kidney beans, drained
    and rinsed
5 cups (1.2 l) Swanson lower sodium, fat-free
    chicken broth
1 tbsp (15 ml) red wine vinegar
1 tsp (5 ml) dried basil leaves
1 tsp (5 ml) white sugar
1 tsp (5 ml) salt
¼ tsp (1 ml) black pepper, freshly ground
8 oz (dry weight) (226 g) ditalini or small shell
    pasta, whole wheat if available
½ cup (120 ml) chopped fresh parsley (or 2 tbsp
    (30ml) dried parsley)
6 tbsp (90 ml) grated parmesan cheese

Heat olive oil over medium heat in a large stockpot.
Choose a pot with a lid because you will cover and
simmer this soup later. Add the minced garlic to the
hot oil in the pot and cook, stirring, for about 30
seconds. Add the onions, carrots, and celery, and
sauté over medium heat until the onions are trans-
parent, about five minutes. Stir frequently. Remove

this concoction to a bowl or plate. The carrots will finish cooking later.

Add the Italian sausage to the stockpot and cook over medium heat for about eight to 12 minutes until fully done, stirring frequently. As it cooks, break the sausage into small chunks using the edge of a rigid turner. A turner is what you would use to flip pancakes, for example.

To the cooked meat in the stockpot, add the sautéed concoction, tomatoes, beans, broth, basil, pepper, salt, vinegar, and sugar. Bring to a boil over high heat, then reduce heat to low and simmer, covered, for an hour. Stir occasionally. Just before serving, add parsley to the pot, and stir once more. If the soup seems too thick, add extra chicken broth or water.

Fill a separate stockpot with water and bring to a boil. Add the pasta and cook according to directions on the box. Then drain the pasta. Mix 1/3 cup (80 ml) pasta and 1 cup (240 ml) soup in a serving bowl, then sprinkle with ½ tbsp (7 ml) grated parmesan cheese. You might enjoy something crunchy with this dish, such as crackers or toast.

Store leftover soup and pasta in separate containers in the refrigerator. The soup tastes just as good, or better, over the next few days. The pasta gets mushy if you mix it into the soup for storage. Add the pasta to the soup just before you eat.
    Servings per batch: 13
    Serving size: 1 cup (240 ml) soup and 1/3 cup (80 ml) cooked pasta
    Box breakdown: ½ grain, 2 veggies, 1 fat (290 cal: 215 from soup, 65 from pasta, 10 from cheese)

Baked Balsamic Honey Mustard Salmon

4 4-oz (113 g) salmon filets
salt and pepper to taste
3 garlic cloves, minced
1 tbsp (15 ml) white wine
1 tbsp (15 ml) Dijon mustard
4 tbsp (60 ml) balsamic vinegar
1 tbsp (15 ml) honey
2 tsp (10 ml) fresh chopped oregano

Preheat the oven to 400°F or 200°C. Line a baking sheet with aluminum foil then spray with PAM cooking spray.

Lightly salt and pepper the fish.

Now prepare the flavorful glaze. Coat a small saucepan with PAM. Sauté the minced garlic over medium heat for about three minutes, until it is soft. Then add and mix the wine, mustard, vinegar, honey, and 1/8 tsp (½ ml) of salt. Simmer uncovered over medium or low-medium heat until slightly thickened, about three minutes. Remove glaze from heat and spoon about half of it into a separate container.

Place the salmon filets on the foil-lined baking sheet, skin-side down, then brush them with the glaze left in the saucepan. Sprinkle oregano on top.

Bake fish in the oven for about 10 to 13 minutes, or until it flakes easily with a fork. Cooking time depends on your oven's actual temperature and thickness of the filet. When done, use a turner to transfer the fish to plates, leaving the skin on the foil if able. Drizzle the glaze from the separate container over the filets with a spoon, or brush it on. Don't use the unwashed brush you used earlier on the raw fish.

Consider serving with a colorful vegetable and whole grain bread. This recipe also works well with halibut, and probably other fish that tend to be a bit bland by themselves.

Servings per batch: 4
Serving size: 1 4-oz (113 g) filet
Box breakdown: 1 protein (225 cal)

SNACKS

Nuts, fruits, cheese, and crackers—see Food Choices and Serving Sizes list for serving sizes. Remember to count them on your Daily Log. Also remember your daily "free" bonus foods that are not logged: three celery stalks and one cup (240 ml) zucchini, radishes, mushrooms, or cucumbers, *and* two cups (480 ml) lettuce, *and* 1 cup (240 ml) parsley. *Or* one sweet pepper. *Or* 3 tbsp (45 ml) diced green chiles.

10
WHAT? ME EXERCISE?

"**A**unt Cheryl, would you take us to Sea World? Please, please, please, please, please?!"

Cheryl was babysitting her eight and 10 year old nieces while their parents were away for the weekend celebrating their wedding anniversary. She stalled for time while trying to come up with an alternative. The kids were bouncing off the walls with energy. Cheryl had enjoyed Sea World 10 years ago, but also remembered the size of the park and how much walking was involved between Shamu and the seal show, and all the exhibits in between.

She was 80 pounds (36 kg) heavier now and knew she couldn't hack it. She fantasized about the kids bolting ahead of her and getting lost in the crowd. What would she tell her brother? "Your daughters were kidnapped because I'm so fat. Sorry."

Mustering all her enthusiasm, she told the children, "Hey! I've got a better idea. Let's go to Chuckie Cheese's instead!" She could safely turn the girls loose there while she sat in a booth reading, eating pizza, and drinking a diet Coke. The girls acquiesced, and off they went. Cheryl wondered if they remembered her huffing, puffing, and sweating her way around the city zoo two years ago.

Shopping at the mall was Cheryl's favorite form of exercise. Uncommonly generous, Cheryl was famous among her friends and relatives for surprising them with unexpected thoughtful tchotchkes as well as more substantial gifts. Walking in from the mall parking lot plus two hours strolling about was a decent workout. But she did it only every couple of weeks. For three hours a week, she volunteered to deliver Meals-On-Wheels, carrying meals into houses and apartments. She spent much more time driving than walking. Of course, she wasn't doing it for the exercise.

Cheryl's only other regular physical activities were housework and walking to and from the parking lot at her job as a librarian. She had hated PE class in school. She never understood why someone would want to exercise when they could spend that time reading, playing cards, relaxing with TV, or playing piano.

By the time she finished gaining those 80 excess pounds (36 kg) of fat between the ages of 20 and 30, she was feeling tired all the time. Her stamina was kaput. She knew 60-year-olds who had more energy than she did. Her knees were aching after the mall trips. She was too young to feel this way! Was there something going on physically other than being overweight? Perhaps diabetes, Chronic Fatigue Syndrome, or a hidden cancer? Most of her relatives were heavy and few of them lived beyond age 65, succumbing to strokes or various cancers. Several relatives had diabetes.

Cheryl's favorite aunt died of cancer at the age of 56. Cheryl, in her early 30s, came to see me six weeks after the funeral. "Doctor Parker, why do I feel so old and tired?" A thorough physical exam and diagnostic lab work revealed only early knee arthritis, mildly elevated blood pressure, and obesity (220 pounds or 100 kg). I was certain that losing the excess weight plus an increase in physical activity would help her immensely. I knew also that convincing her, much less altering her behavior, would be an uphill battle. But I was prepared to help her win it.

EXERCISE AND WEIGHT LOSS

Exercise is overrated as a pathway to major weight loss. Sure, a physically inactive young man with only five or 10 pounds (2 to 4 kg) to lose might be able to do it simply by starting an exercise program. That doesn't work nearly as well for women. The problem is that exercise stimulates appetite, so any calories burned by exercise tend to be counteracted by increased food consumption, whether consciously or not.

Have you seen TV's "Biggest Loser" show? Contestants do lose a huge amount of weight through a combination of extreme amounts of exercise (several hours daily) and major calorie restriction. Participants are pulled out of their usual living situation and put in a supportive yet highly competitive environment. They're competing for their 15 minutes of TV fame, as well as substantial money: $250,000 in the U.S. version. If you can replicate that setting, exercise does indeed help with weight loss. But that's an unrealistic scenario for most of us.

For the average person wanting to lose excess weight, regular exercise may contribute about 10% to a successful effort, with the other 90% coming from the eating end of the equation.

If you know from past experience that exercise helps you lose weight, then work it.

On the other hand, what's the role of exercise in maintenance of weight loss? In other words, does exercise help prevent weight regain? Yes. Surveys of successful long-term "losers" consistently show that regular exercise is strongly linked to prevention of regain. We're looking at 45 to 60 minutes of exercise on most days of the week.

If you're going to invest that much of your time, you'll be glad to know that regular physical activity has lots of other beneficial effects.

EXERCISE BENEFITS

DEATH PREVENTION AND POSTPONEMENT

As many as 250,000 deaths per year in the United States (approximately 12% of the total) are attributable to a lack of regular physical activity. We know now that regular physical activity can prevent a significant number of these deaths. Exercise induces metabolic changes that lessen the impact of, or prevent altogether, several major illnesses, such as high blood pressure, coronary artery disease, diabetes, and obesity. There are also psychological benefits.

PHYSICAL FITNESS AND AEROBIC POWER

To understand how exercise prevents and postpones death, we need to first define exercise, physical fitness, and aerobic power.

Exercise is planned, structured, and repetitive bodily movement done to improve or maintain physical fitness.

Physical fitness is a set of attributes that relate to your ability to perform physical activity. These attributes include resting heart rate, blood pressure at rest and during exercise, lung capacity, body composition (weight in relation to height, percentage of body fat and muscle, bone structure), and aerobic power.

Aerobic power takes some explanation. Muscles perform their work by contracting, which shortens the muscles, pulling on attached tendons or bones. The resultant movement is physical activity. Muscle contraction requires energy, which is obtained from chemical reactions that use oxygen. Oxygen from the air we breathe is delivered to muscle tissue by the lungs, heart, and blood vessels. The ability of the cardiopulmonary system to transport oxygen from the atmosphere to the working muscles is called maximal oxygen uptake, or aerobic power. It's the primary factor limiting performance of muscular activity.

Aerobic power is commonly measured by having a person perform progressively more difficult exercise on a treadmill or bicycle to the point of exhaustion. The treadmill test starts at a walking pace and gets faster and steeper every few minutes. The longer the subject can last on the treadmill, the greater his aerobic power. A large aerobic power is one of the most reliable indicators of good physical fitness. It's cultivated through consistent, repetitive physical activity.

Higher levels of physical fitness are linked to lower rates of death primarily from cancer and cardiovascular disease (e.g., heart attacks and stroke). What's more, moving from a lower to a higher level of fitness also prolongs life, even for people over 60. How do you get from a lower to higher level of fitness? Start an exercise program or intensify and existing one.

METABOLIC EFFECTS OF EXERCISE

Where does the fat go when you lose weight dieting? Chemical reactions convert it to energy, water, and carbon dioxide, which weigh less than the fat. Most of your energy supply is used to fuel basic life-maintaining physiologic processes at rest, referred to as resting or basal metabolism. Basal metabolic rate (BMR) is expressed as calories per kilogram of body weight per hour.

The major determinants of BMR are age, sex, and the body's relative proportions of muscle and fat. Heredity plays a lesser role. Energy not used for basal metabolism is either stored as fat or converted by the muscles to physical activity. Most of us use about 70% of our energy supply for basal metabolism and 30% for physical activity. Those who exercise regularly and vigorously may expend 40–60% of their calorie intake doing physical activity. Excess energy not used in resting metabolism or physical activity is stored as fat.

Insulin, remember, is the main hormone converting that excess energy into fat; and carbohydrates are the major cause of insulin release by the pancreas. Excessive carbohydrate consumption in particular drives the imbalance towards overweight, via insulin's fat-storing properties.

In terms of losing weight, the most important metabolic effect of exercise is that it turns fat into weightless energy. We see that weekly on TV's "Biggest Loser" show; participants exercise a huge amount.

Physical activity alone as a weight-loss method isn't very effective. But there are several other reasons to recommend exercise to those wishing to lose weight. Exercise counteracts the decrease in basal metabolic rate seen with some calorie-restricted diets. In some folks, exercise temporarily reduces appetite (but others note the opposite effect). While caloric restriction during dieting can diminish your sense of energy and vitality, exercise typically does the opposite. Many dieters, especially those on low-calorie poorly designed diets, lose lean tissue (such as muscle and water) in addition to fat. This isn't desirable over the long run. Exercise counteracts the tendency to lose muscle mass while nevertheless modestly facilitating fat loss.

Again, how much does exercise contribute to most successful weight-loss efforts? Only about 10% on average. The other 90% is from food restriction.

FOUNTAIN OF YOUTH

Regular exercise is a demonstrable "fountain of youth." Peak aerobic power (or fitness) naturally diminishes by 50% between young adulthood and age 65. In other words, as age advances even a light physical task becomes fatiguing if it is sustained over time. By the age of 75 or 80, many of us depend on others for help with the ordinary tasks of daily living, such as housecleaning and grocery shopping. Regular exercise increases fitness (aerobic power) by 15–20% in middle-aged and older men and women, the equivalent of a 10–20 year reduction in biological age! This prolongation of self-sufficiency improves quality of life.

HEART HEALTH

Exercise helps control multiple cardiac (heart attack) risk factors: obesity, high cholesterol, elevated blood pressure, high triglycerides, and diabetes.

Regular aerobic activity tends to lower LDL cholesterol, the "bad cholesterol." Jogging 10 or 12 miles a week, or the equivalent amount of other exercise, increases HDL cholesterol ("good cholesterol") substantially.

Aerobic exercise done on a regular basis lowers blood pressure by 8–11 points (mmHg), That's equivalent to many blood pressure medications, without the expense and side effects of drugs.

Exercise increases heart muscle efficiency and blood flow to the heart. For the person who has already had a heart attack, regular physical activity decreases the incidence of fatal recurrence by 20–30% and adds an extra two or three years of life, on average.

EFFECT ON DIABETES

Eighty-five percent of type 2 diabetics are over-weight or obese. It's not just a random association. Obesity contributes heavily to most cases of type 2 diabetes, particularly in those predisposed by heredity. Insulin is the key that allows bloodstream sugar (glucose) into cells for utilization as energy, thus keeping blood sugar from reaching dangerously high levels. Overweight bodies produce plenty of insulin, often more than average. The problem in overweight diabetics is that the cells are no longer sensitive to insulin's effect. Weight loss and exercise independently return insulin sensitivity towards normal. Many diabetics can improve their condition through sensible exercise and weight management.

MISCELLANEOUS BENEFITS

In case you need more reasons to start or keep exercising, consider the following additional benefits: 1) enhanced immune function, 2) stronger bones, 3) preservation and improvement of flexibility, 4) diminished premenstrual bloating, breast tenderness, and mood changes, 5) reduced incidence of dementia, 6) less trouble with constipation, 7) better ability to handle stress, 8) less trouble with insomnia, 9) improved self-esteem, 10) enhanced sense of well-being, with less anxiety and depression, 11) higher perceived level of energy, and 12) prevention of weight regain.

EXERCISE RECOMMENDATIONS

Now that you know the health benefits of exercise, it's a little easier to understand those crazy people you see jogging at 6 a.m. in below-freezing weather. I'm sure you're ready to join them tomorrow morning. Right?

Here's some good news. Most people following both the Ketogenic and Advanced Mediterranean Diets are able to lose excess weight and improve glucose control without starting an exercise program. Many—but certainly not all—will be able to maintain a stable, reasonable weight long-term without ongoing exercise. However, for the reasons already outlined, I recommend you start a physical activity program eventually. If following the Advanced Mediterranean program, start now.

I must warn you that athletic individuals who perform vigorous exercise should expect a deterioration in performance levels during the first three to four weeks of any very-low-carb ketogenic diet, including the Ketogenic Mediterranean Diet. The body needs that time to adjust to burning mostly fat for fuel rather than carbohydrate.

Also, competitive weight-lifters or other anaerobic athletes (e.g., sprinters) may be hampered by the low muscle glycogen stores that accompany ketogenic diets. They need more carbohydrates for high-level performance.

HOW MUCH EXERCISE?

All I'm asking you to do is aerobic activity, such as walk briskly (3–4 mph or 4.8–6.4 km/h) for 30 minutes most days of the week, and do some muscle-strengthening exercises three times a week. This amount of exercise will get you most of the documented health benefits. It's OK if you want to wait until you've lost some of your excess weight, but I probably wouldn't.

Keep reading to find out if exercise would be a bad idea for you

The U.S. Centers for Disease Control and Prevention recommends at least 150 minutes per week of moderate-intensity aerobic activity (e.g., brisk walking) and muscle-strengthening activity at least twice a week, OR 75 minutes per week of vigorous-intensity aerobic activity (e.g., running or jogging) plus muscle-strengthening activity at least twice a week. The muscle-strengthening activity should work all the major muscle groups: legs, hips, back, abdomen, chest, shoulders, and arms.

Please note that you don't have to run marathons (26.2 miles) or compete in the Ironman Triathlon to earn the health benefits of exercise. However, if health promotion and disease prevention are your goals, plan on a lifetime commitment to regular physical activity.

Don't feel bad if you haven't been exercising; you're not alone. Twenty-five percent of U.S. adults are completely sedentary. Only two or three of every 10 Americans are active enough to gain all the health benefits of exercise.

STRENGTH TRAINING

What's "strength training"? It's also called muscle-strengthening activity, resistance training, weight training, and resistance exercise. Examples include lifting weights, work with resistance bands, digging, shoveling, yoga, push-ups, chin-ups, and other exercises that use your body weight or other loads for resistance.

Strength training three times a week increases your strength and endurance, allows you to sculpt your body to an extent, and counteracts the loss of lean body mass (muscle) so often seen during efforts to lose excess weight. It also helps maintain your functional abilities as you age. For example, it's a major chore for many 80-year-olds to climb a flight of stairs, carry in a bag of groceries from the car, or vacuum a house. Strength training helps maintain these abilities that youngsters take for granted.

According to the U.S. Centers for Disease Control and Prevention: "To gain health benefits, muscle-strengthening activities need to be done to the point where it's hard for you to do another repetition without help. A repetition is one complete movement of an activity, like lifting a weight or doing a sit-up. Try to do 8–12 repetitions per activity that count as 1 set. Try to do at least 1 set of muscle-strengthening activities, but to gain even more benefits, do 2 or 3 sets."

If this is starting to sound like Greek to you, consider instruction by a personal trainer at a local gym or health club. That's a good investment for anyone unfamiliar with strength training, in view of its great benefits and the potential harm or waste of time from doing it wrong. If cost is an issue, the YMCA or YWCA may be less expensive. Alternatives to a personal trainer would be help from an experienced friend or instructional DVD. If you're determined to go it alone, Internet resources may help, but be careful. Consider "Growing Stronger: Strength Training for Older Adults" (http://www.cdc.gov/physicalactivity/downloads/growing_stronger.pdf). Doug Robb's blog, HealthHabits, is a wonderful source of strength training advice (http://www.healthhabits.ca/).

In 2011, I made a serious commitment to Mark Verstegen's Core Performance workout program. Done in the privacy of my home, it combines strength training, cardio (aerobics), flexibility, and balance training. I'm very happy with results. Check out his book at Amazon.com.

Current strength training techniques are much different than what you remember from high school 30 years ago—modern methods are better. Some of the latest research suggests that strength training may be even more beneficial than aerobic exercise.

AEROBIC ACTIVITY

What's "aerobic activity"? Just about anything that mostly makes you huff and puff. In other words, get short of breath to some degree. Examples are brisk walking, swimming, golf (pulling a cart or carrying clubs), lawn work, painting, home repair, racket sports and table tennis, house cleaning, leisurely canoeing, jogging, bicycling, jumping rope, and skiing. The possibilities are endless. A leisurely stroll in the shopping mall doesn't qualify, unless that makes you short of breath. Don't laugh: that *is* a workout for many who are obese.

But which aerobic physical activity is best? Glad you asked!

The most important criterion is that it be pleasant for you. If not outright fun, it should be often enjoyable and always tolerable.

Your exercise of choice should also be available year-round, affordable, safe, and utilize large muscle groups. The greater mass and number of muscles used, the more calories you will burn, which is important if you're trying to lose weight or prevent gain. Compare tennis playing with sitting in a chair squeezing a tennis ball repetitively. The tennis player burns calories much faster. Your largest muscles are in your legs, so consider walking, biking, many team sports, ski machines, jogging, treadmill, swimming, water aerobics, stationary cycling, stairsteppers, tennis, volleyball, roller-skating, rowing, jumping rope, and yard work.

The following table lists the average number of calories burned during a few types of aerobic physical activity (aka "cardio") for a person weighing 150 pounds (68 kg). Heavier people would tend to expend more calories. Calories burned during your particular physical activity are difficult to predict and measure. But don't choose an activity just because it burns lots of calories. That's a certain path to injury or quick burn out. Then you won't be exercising at all.

Calories Expended by a 150-Pound (68 kg) Person
in 15 Minutes of Various Activities

Activity	Calories
Walking 2 mph (3.2 km/h)	60
Walking 3 mph (4.8 km/h)	75
Walking 4 mph (6.4 km/h)	100
Bicycling 6 mph (9.7 km/h)	65
Bicycling 12 mph (19 km/h)	100
Tennis, singles	100
Jogging 5.5 mph (8.9 km/h)	160

| Jumping rope | 160 |
| Cross-country skiing | 160 |

Walking is "just what the doctor ordered" for many people. It's readily available, affordable, usually safe, and requires little instruction. If it's too hot, too cold, or rainy outside, you can do it in a mall, gymnasium, or health club.

Another option is instructional exercise DVDs, often featuring either a celebrity or prominent fitness trainer. Many of these programs require only a pair of sneakers and loose clothing. Others include the option of using inexpensive equipment, such as light hand-held weights.

If exercise videos sound appealing, consider one of these: *Walk Away the Pounds—Walk Strong*, by Leslie Sansone; *Tighter Assets With Tamilee: Weight Loss & Cardio*, by Tamilee Webb; *Burn & Firm—Circuit Training*, by Karen Voight; *Minna Optimizer—Balanced Blend*, by Minna Lessig; *Personal Training System*, by Denise Austin; *Timesaver—Lift Weights to Lose Weight (volumes 1 & 2), Super Slimdown Circuit, and Functionally Fit—Peak Fat Burning*, by Kathy Smith. Search for these titles at Amazon.com, where you can read reviews of them by actual users. Although many of these are designed for weight loss, you'll get a good workout even if you're at a healthy weight. Several of them also feature strength training.

Another fun option for indoor aerobic exercise is Dance Dance Revolution by Konami. Perhaps you've seen a version of this video game in an arcade. You must use a video game console, such as a PlayStation or Xbox, and the Dance Dance Revolution Controller along with your TV screen. The controller is a 32 inch by 36 inch (81 x 91 cm) floor pad partitioned into several large squares. The TV screen shows you which squares to step on in sequence as the music plays, and you rack up points for accurate timing and foot placement. If you enjoy moving to music, it's more fun than I can describe.

The latest indoor computerized exercise gadgets are the Kinect for Microsoft's Xbox 360, the PlayStation Move, and Wii Fit. Check'em out.

MAKE IT A HABIT

The main objective at this point is to make regular physical activity a habit. Establishment of a habit requires frequent repetition over at least two or three months, regardless of the weather, whether you feel like it or not. Over time the chosen activity becomes part of your identity.

PRACTICAL POINTS

To avoid injury and burn out, begin your exercise program slowly and increase the intensity of your effort only every two or three weeks. Your body needs time to adjust to its new workload, but it will indeed adjust. Enhance your enjoyment with proper attire, equipment, and instruction, if needed. Use a portable radio or digital music system like an iPod or Zune if you tend to get bored exercising.

The "buddy system" works well for many of my patients: agree with a friend that you'll meet regularly for walking, jogging, whatever. If you know your buddy is counting on you to show up at the park at 7 a.m., it may be just the motivation you need to get you out of bed. Others just can't handle such regimentation and enjoy the flexibility and independence of solitary activity.

If you like to socialize, join a health club or sports team. Large cities have organized clubs that promote a wide range of physical activities. Find your niche.

Don't be afraid to try something new. Expect some disappointment and failed experiments. Learn and grow from adversity and failure. Put a lot of thought into your choice of activity. Avoid built-in barriers. If you live in Florida you won't have much opportunity for cross-country skiing. If joining a health club is a financial strain, walk instead. Perhaps pick different activities for cold and warm weather. Or do several types of exercise to avoid boredom.

In summary, formation of the exercise habit requires forethought, repetition, and commitment. You must schedule time for physical activity. Make it a priority. Hundreds of my couch potato patients have done it, and I'm sure you can, too. I've seen 40-year-old unathletic, uncoordinated barnacles start exercising and run marathons two years later. (A marathon is 26.2 miles or 42.2 km.)

MEDICAL CLEARANCE

To protect you from injury, I recommend that you obtain "medical clearance" from a personal physician before starting an exercise program. A physician is in the best position to determine if your plans are safe for you, thereby avoiding complications such as injury and death. Nevertheless, most adults can start a moderate-intensity exercise program with little risk. An example of moderate intensity would be walking briskly (3–4 mph or 4.8–6.4 km/h) for 30 minutes daily.

Men over 40 and women over 50 who anticipate a more vigorous program should consult a physician to ensure safety. The physician may well recommend diagnostic blood work, an electrocardiogram (heart electrical tracing), and an exercise stress test (often on a treadmill). The goal is not to generate fees for the doctor, but to find the occasional person for whom exercise will be dangerous, if not fatal. Those who drop dead at the start of a vigorous exercise program often have an undiagnosed heart condition, such as blockages in the arteries that supply the heart muscle. The doctor will also look for other dangerous undiagnosed "silent" conditions, such as leaky heart valves, hereditary heart conditions, aneurysms, extremely high blood pressure, and severe diabetes.

Regardless of age, other folks who may benefit from a medical consultation before starting an exercise program include those with known high blood pressure, high cholesterol, joint problems (e.g., arthritis, degenerated discs), neurologic problems, poor circulation, diabetes, lung disease, or any other significant chronic medical condition. Also be sure to check with a doctor first if you've been experiencing chest pains, palpitations, dizziness, fainting spells, headaches, frequent urination, or any unusual symptoms (particularly during exertion).

Physicians, physiatrists, physical therapists, and exercise physiologists can also be helpful in the design of a safe, effective exercise program for those with established chronic medical conditions.

REALISTIC GOALS

Sustained physical activity requires that your heart pump blood to the lungs and then to the exercising muscles. The muscles extract oxygen, sugar, and other nutrients for use in chemical reactions that enable the muscle to keep moving (contracting). To say that someone is physically fit simply means that the heart easily pumps a large volume of blood and the muscles extract and use nutrients very efficiently. The heart, after all, is just a hollow muscle that pumps blood. If you stimulate your heart muscle through exercise, it will become more powerful and able to pump more blood. Regular sessions of physical activity increase the metabolic efficiency and power of your other muscles, too. There are various degrees of fitness, with professional and Olympic athletes at the extreme upper end.

GETTING STARTED

I've had otherwise healthy overweight patients so "out of shape" that walking 20 yards (18 meters) to the mailbox was a real chore. They were tired and panting when they got to the mailbox and had to rest a bit before returning to the house. These folks are habitually sedentary and dramatically overweight. But you need not feel too sorry for them. After starting and maintaining an exercise program, these unfit people achieve the greatest degree of improvement in fitness levels. They make more progress, and faster, than those who begin with a greater level of fitness.

The way to achieve aerobic fitness is to regularly challenge your large muscles to perform sustained physical activity. "Regularly" means at least three days a week, if not daily. I do recommend at least one day of rest weekly.

Left alone, your muscles don't want to do much other than just get you through your day comfortably, without effort or aching or cramps. You must challenge them to do more, work a bit harder, tolerate a little aching. You will know you are challenging them during exercise when you perceive that mild to moderate effort is required to keep the activity going. You should be mildly short of breath, perhaps even perspiring lightly, yet still able to converse. "Sustained" physical activity means at least 30 minutes in a day. Most people find it a better use of their time to exercise for 30 minutes continuously rather than break it up into five or 10 minutes here and there.

Discontinuous activity (e.g., 10 minutes thrice daily) probably is just as good. If you think about it, there are many easy ways to increase your discontinuous physical activity. Consider taking the stairs instead of the elevator, parking far from the supermarket or workplace doors, walking the golf course instead of riding a cart.

If you're starting out in poor shape, you won't be able to do 30 minutes of any exercise without adverse effects. Don't even try. The worst thing you could do at this point is injure yourself or have such a horrible experience that you give up entirely. Thirty minutes of almost daily activity is your goal to achieve over the next four to 12 months. Moderate to high levels of fitness will take you six to 24 months. The most important thing when getting started is to exercise at least a little, five to 10 minutes, on most days of the week. And don't overdo it in terms of intensity. Start low, go slow. After three months, exercise will be a habit. Prolongation of your exercise sessions will be easy as your amazing body responds gradually to the workload through the process called physical conditioning.

If walking 30 minutes daily is too hard for you at first, try walking just an extra 10 or 20 minutes daily. If you can do that but it's a bit of a strain, gradually (every two weeks) increase your walking time by five minutes daily until you're up to 30 minutes. Average walking pace is 2 mph (3.2 km/h). Once you can comfortably handle 30 minutes daily, the next step is to increase your walking pace to 3 or 4 mph (4.8–6.4 km/h) for the entire 30 minutes. Four mph (6.4 km/h) is definitely a brisk walk. It's difficult for many people to sustain over 30 minutes until they work up to it gradually. This is often done by walking at two paces, normal and brisk, during an exercise session. You might walk five minutes at normal pace, then five minutes briskly, alternating every five minutes until the session is over. Every two to four weeks, you can increase the minutes of brisk pace and taper off the normal pace. You're able to do this easily because your level of fitness is increasing.

I'm asking you to walk briskly (3–4 mph or 4.8–6.4 km/h) for 30 minutes most days of the week. This brisk pace burns roughly 200 calories per session, in case you're wondering. If you eat a 400-calorie muffin, it provides enough energy for a one-hour brisk walk. If you don't burn the muffin calories as exercise or basal metabolism, they'll turn into body fat. (But you're not eating muffins anymore, are you?!)

If you prefer physical activity other than walking, the general rule is to start slowly and gradually increase your effort (intensity) until you're up to about

30 minutes of moderate-intensity exercise most days of the week. Start low, go slow.

IF YOU ARE MARKEDLY OBESE

The more overweight you are, the harder it will be to exercise. At some point even light exercise becomes impossible. Average-height women tipping the scales at about 280 pounds (127 kg) and men at 360 pounds (164 kg) aren't going to be able to jog around the block, much less run a marathon. These weights are 100% over ideal or healthy levels. An actual "exercise program" probably won't be possible until some weight is lost simply through very-low-carb eating, calorie restriction, or bariatric surgery. The initial exercise goal for you may just be to get moving through activities of daily living and perhaps brief walks, and calisthenics while sitting in a chair.

Markedly obese people who aren't up to the aforementioned extreme weights can usually tolerate a low-intensity physical activity program. At 50% over ideal weight, an average-height woman of 210 pounds (95 kg) is carrying 70 excess pounds (32 kg) of fat. Her male counterpart lugs around 90 pounds (41 kg) of unnecessary fat. This weight burden causes dramatic breathlessness and fatigue upon exertion, and makes the joints and muscles more susceptible to aching and injury. If you're skinny, just imagine trying to walk or run a mile carrying a standard five-gallon (19 liter) water cooler bottle, which weighs only 43 pounds (19.5 kg) when full. The burden of excess fat makes it quite difficult to exercise.

If you're markedly obese, several tricks will enhance your exercise success. I want you to avoid injury, frustration, and burn out. Start with light activity for only 10 or 15 minutes, gradually increase session length (e.g., by two to four minutes every two to four weeks) and increase exercise intensity only after several months. Your joints and muscles may appreciate easy, low-impact exercises such as stationary cycling, walking, swimming, and pool calisthenics/water aerobics. You may also benefit from the advice of a personal fitness trainer arranged through a health club, gym, or YMCA/YWCA. Check out several health clubs before you join. Some of them are primarily meat markets for beautiful slender yuppies. You may feel more comfortable in a gym that welcomes and caters to overweight people. Hospitals are increasingly developing fitness centers with obese orthopedic, heart, and diabetic patients in mind.

PEDOMETERS

A pedometer attached to your waistband may help motivate you by tracking total step count, distance traveled, and calories burned. Reliable pedometers cost $20 to $30 (US) and are available at sporting goods stores, sports shoe stores, and via the Internet.

Consumer Reports magazine in February, 2009, reviewed pedometers and their #1 Best Buy recommendation was the Omron HJ 112, which you can clip to your belt or waistband, or carry in your purse. It's available for around $15–30 (US). No.2 was the Accusplit AE 170 XLG ($30–35), which I own and recommend. The Accusplit AE 170 may be just as good. The only difference I see is that you can enter your specific goals into the XLG.

259

The Omron HIP (HJ 150, $20) is also very popular and probably the simplest one to use of the three mentioned. The guys at Obesity Panacea blog (Peter Janiszewski and Travis Saunders, both Ph.D.s) recommend the Omron HJ-303 ($35), which you can carry in your pocket instead of clipped to your waistband.

Sedentary people walk 2,000–4,000 steps daily as they go about their lives. Your goal now is 8,000–10,000 daily steps. Ten-thousand steps covers about 5 miles (8 kilometers). Appropriate comfortable shoes are well worth the money.

A high-tech alternative to a pedometer is Nike+ (Nike Plus), which is geared more toward runners.

TARGET HEART RATE

One rough way to gauge whether you're working hard enough during exercise is to monitor your heart rate, also known as pulse. Subtract your age from 220. The result is your theoretical maximum heart rate in beats per minute. Your heart rate goal, or target, during sustained aerobic exercise is a pulse that is 60 to 80% of your theoretical maximum pulse. For example: maximum heart rate for a 40-year-old is 180 (220 - 40 = 180), so the target heart rate zone during exercise is between 108 and 144 (60 to 80% of 180). Exceeding the upper end of the target zone is usually too uncomfortable to be sustainable. Exercise heart rates below the target zone suggest you're not working hard enough to reap the full long-term benefits of aerobic exercise.

Here's how to determine your pulse. After five or 10 minutes of exercise, stop moving and place the tips of your first two fingers lightly over the pulse spot inside your wrist just below the base of your thumb. Count the pulsations for 15 seconds and multiply the number by four. The result is your pulse or heart rate. It will take some practice to find those pulsations coming from your radial artery. If you can't find it, ask a nurse or doctor for help.

Like all rules-of-thumb, this target heart rate zone isn't always an accurate gauge of cardiovascular workout intensity. For instance, it's of very little use in people taking drugs called beta blockers, which keep a lid on heart rate.

As you become more fit, you'll notice that you have to work harder to get your heart rate up to a certain level. This is a sure sign that your heart and muscles are responding to your challenge. You may also want to monitor your resting heart rate taken in the morning before you get out of bed. Unfit, sedentary people have resting pulses of 60 to 90. Athletes are more often in the 40s or low 50s. Their hearts have become more efficient and just don't need to beat as often to get the job done.

As you become more fit, you'll also notice that you have more energy overall and it's easier to move about and handle physical workloads. You'll feel more relaxed and have a sense of accomplishment. Expect these benefits eight to 12 weeks after starting a regular exercise program.

EXERCISE EQUIPMENT

You don't need to spend hundreds of dollars for new exercise equipment. Check Craig's List (or similar) and the classified ads of your newspaper for big discounts on "pre-owned" motorized treadmills, stationary bicycles, rowing machines, dumbbells, weight machines, and other devices. Avoid the exclusive abdominal muscle exercisers. Remember, you want to exercise the large muscles. You may have great "abs" but no one will know it if they're camouflaged behind three inches of fat.

EXERCISE WITH JOINT AND BACK PAIN

Painful lower limb joints and chronic or recurrent back pain are an exercise barrier to many people. Those affected should consult a physician for a diagnosis, treatment, and advice on appropriate physical activity. If the physician isn't sure about an exercise prescription, consultation with an orthopedist, physiatrist, or physical therapist should be helpful. Generally, weight-bearing on bad joints should be minimized by doing pool calisthenics, stationary cycling, swimming, etc. Use your imagination. Particularly bothersome joints may not tolerate exercise, if ever, until weight is lost by other methods, such as very-low-carb eating (see the Ketogenic Mediterranean Diet). Light to moderate exercise actually reduces the pain and disability of knee degenerative arthritis. The effect is modest and comes with a small risk of injury such as bone fracture, cartilage tears, arthritis flare, and soft tissue strain.

SUMMARY

Again, the goal is 30 minutes of brisk walking most days of the week, plus strength training three days a week. Walking faster or longer, and more vigorous types of exercise, might help you lose weight faster and achieve higher levels of fitness. But committing much more time and energy to exercise just isn't going to happen for many folks. Fortunately, most of the general health benefits of an active lifestyle are gained by a simple 30-minute daily brisk walk or similar aerobic exercise.

Exercise isn't for everybody, and not everybody responds to exercise with good weight management and becoming shapelier. Your heredity limits your response to exercise to an uncertain extent. I challenge you to define your limits by putting your body through the paces.

You may still be able to control your weight even if you don't exercise, particularly if you avoid the fattening carbohydrates like concentrated sugars and refined starches.

If you can't manage regular physical activity during your period of weight loss, at least give it another chance as you move into your maintenance-of-weight-loss phase. Regular exercise is the single best predictor of successful long-term weight management.

Exercise may not be easy, it may not be popular, it may not be what you want to hear, but it's the right thing to do.

You met my patient, Cheryl, at the start of this chapter. She had gained 80 pounds (36 kg) between the ages of 20 and 30. Cheryl had always been sedentary and had little enthusiasm for starting an exercise program at this point in her life. I told her that regular physical activity would greatly improve her long-range health outlook and her odds of regaining weight once she lost it. She was disappointed, but confirmed my position by doing her own research at the library where she worked.

Cheryl readily learned how to control her caloric intake with the Advanced Mediterranean Diet. We discussed various exercise options. She chose to join a gym and work out on a stationary bike and stair-stepper machine. She listened to audio books and talk radio through earphones while exercising, to help her pass the time. Simple analgesics relieved her minor knee discomfort. After six months, she transitioned to outdoor walking. At that point she was 30 pounds (14 kg) lighter, so her knees quit aching. On rainy days she worked out indoors using instructional exercise DVDs.

Over the course of a year, Cheryl lost 65 pounds (30 kg). A combination of weight loss, exercise, and diet brought her blood pressure down into the normal range without drug therapy. Her knees appreciated the lighter load. And she had the energy and stamina of a healthy 30-something woman not burdened by 65 pounds (30 kg) of excess fat. Finally, Cheryl reduced her chances of developing the cancer, strokes, and diabetes that afflicted so many of her relatives.

KEY POINTS

- Lack of regular exercise causes preventable deaths.
- Increasing your level of fitness can reduce your risk of death from cardiovascular disease and cancer.
- The energy you eat, minus the energy you burn in metabolism and activity, determines your change in body fat.
- Energy expenditure is a combination of basal metabolism and physical activity.
- Exercise turns body fat into weightless energy, unless you eat too much.

- Once you lose your excess weight, regular exercise will greatly enhance your success in keeping the weight off.
- Exercise is a demonstrable fountain of youth.

I do not like broccoli. And I haven't liked it since I was a little kid and my mother made me eat it. And I'm President of the United States and I'm not going to eat anymore broccoli.
— George H.W. Bush, 1990

11

Long-Term Maintenance and Prevention of Weight Regain

Reaccumulation of lost body fat is the most problematic area in the field of weight management. You may have heard that "diets don't work," but they do. Many different programs work short-term, if "work" is defined as loss of five, 10, or more pounds (two, four, or more kg) while you adhere to the program for several weeks or months. The problem is that the lost pounds usually return. You get bored with the diet, or your willpower flags, or the diet simply stops working, the transition from weight loss to maintenance is unclear, you just feel too bad to go on, you lose your commitment, you take a job as a taste tester for Baskin-Robbins Ice Cream, or whatever.

Most diets ultimately fail in the long run simply because people go back to their old habits.

FINALLY AT GOAL WEIGHT

For purposes of further discussion, I'll assume that you've already lost weight down to your goal and now must focus on staying thereabouts from here on out.

Finally down to your goal! A grand accomplishment! You've got a new wardrobe, or the old clothes fit again. You have more energy and feel younger. Maybe you cured or improved some health problems. Perhaps you're getting more attention from the opposite sex.

The scientific name for humans is *Homo sapiens.* Sapiens is from the Latin sapere, which means "to be wise." Wisdom is the ability to make correct judgments and decisions. Undoubtedly, your success at weight loss required correct judgments and decisions. You're not done yet. You'll need sustained wisdom to avoid weight regain.

Be wise about this especially: you can never again eat all you want, whatever you want, whenever you want, over sustained periods of time.

Now that you've reached your goal weight, you must restrain yourself on a daily basis. Think about it. You became overweight because you didn't watch what you ate. Inadequate exercise may well have contributed, too. You can't go back to your old ways. Reject this advice, and you have a 100 percent chance of regaining your lost weight.

Remember the Energy Balance Equation?

Calorie Intake minus Calories Burned
= Change in Body Fat

You've been able to lose fat weight because you ate less energy (calories) than your body required for metabolism and physical activity. Your body remedied the energy deficit by converting fat into energy. A pound (454 g) of fat contains 3,500 calories of energy. If you lost a pound (454 g) per week, your body on average converted 500 calories of body fat daily into energy (7 days x 500 calories = 3,500 calories = 1 pound or 454 g of fat).

Now that you're at your goal weight and want to stay there, you need to add some calories back into the equation. Add the calories by eating more food, exercising less, or a combination of the two. But if you add back too many calories, you'll regain weight. Carbohydrate calories are particularly effective at packing the fat back on, because they stimulate release of the fat-building hormone, insulin. The fattening carbohydrates typically are concentrated sugars and refined starches.

KETOGENIC MEDITERRANEAN DIET: TRANSITION TO MAINTENANCE PHASE

If you've been following the Advanced Mediterranean Diet, this section isn't for you. Go to the next major section about nine pages ahead.

I'll assume readers of this section have been following the Ketogenic Mediterranean Diet (KMD) for at least a couple weeks, if not for several months or more. I recommend at least 8–12 weeks.

At this point you're ready for a change either because you've reached your weight-loss goal or you want a greater variety of carbohydrates (carbs). Stay familiar with the KMD because it's the foundation for everything that will follow. You're not really done with it; you're adding to it, moving from a very-low-carb diet to the Low-Carb Mediterranean Diet.

The Low-Carb Mediterranean Diet (LCMD) loosens up on food restrictions and introduces additional carbohydrates as long as weight management doesn't deteriorate.

Perhaps you've been losing weight steadily with the KMD and are not yet at your goal weight but crave more food variety. Many continue to lose excess weight with the Low-Carb Mediterranean Diet, although it tends to be easier with the KMD. If weight loss stalls, just return to the KMD.

Alternatively, perhaps you're simply interested in eating more of the plant-based foods linked to the health benefits of the traditional Mediterranean diet.

The KMD may be perfectly healthy long-term; we just don't know for sure. I think it is. On the other hand, there is at least some evidence that additional carbohydrates, as in the Low-Carb Mediterranean Diet, may be even healthier. For example, some scientific studies link fruit and vegetable consumption with lower rates of cancer, stroke, and coronary heart disease. [Other studies find no benefit.] Whole grain consumption is associated with lower rates of cardiovascular disease, including heart attacks and strokes. Legumes (such as beans and peas) are a great source of fiber to counteract the constipation common with very-low-carb diets like the KMD. Additional fruits and vegetables might contribute to longevity, prevent dementia, and help preserve vision by preventing macular degeneration.

And some added carbohydrates may just plain taste good!

My primary goal with the KMD and LCMD is to reap the health benefits of a Mediterranean style diet while not allowing too many fattening carbs that sabotage weight-management efforts.

OVERVIEW OF THE LOW-CARB MEDITERRANEAN DIET

You've been eating 20 to 30 grams of carbohydrate daily on the KMD. Now you're going to increase to 40–100 grams daily, gradually adding carbs that may have beneficial effects on health and longevity. Adding excessive carbs will lead inevitably to regain of lost weight, or a stall in weight-loss progress.

Also note that excessive consumption of easily digested carbs is linked to future diabetes, heart disease, and gallbladder disease, at least in women. So we may as well aim for reasonable carb restriction.

If you're not at your goal weight already, adding too many carb grams now will impair your ability to convert your body fat into energy. Eat too many carbs, and your body will use them for the energy it needs rather than your body's fat. You may well continue to lose weight eating 40, 60, or 100 grams a day, but maybe not. Remember, the typical American adult eats about 275 grams of carb daily, and two thirds of us are overweight or obese.

LET'S GET STARTED ON LCMD!

So, what healthy carbs are we going to add to the Ketogenic Mediterranean Diet, transforming it into the Low-Carb Mediterranean Diet? Fruits, more vegetables (including starchy ones), legumes, yogurt and other dairy products, and whole grains.

To avoid carb overdose and loss of weight control, we're adding back carbs incrementally and slowly.

I've divided the new carbohydrates into groups and specified a serving size for each source of carbs. Each serving has about 7.5 grams of digestible carbohydrate.

What you do next is add one daily carb serving from the list of Carb Groups and Serving Sizes in Table 11.1 (listed a few pages ahead) and see what happens with your weight over the next week. This is not one carb serving on Monday, two on Tuesday, three on Wednesday, etc. It's seven new carb servings per week, one on each day.

Continue to weigh yourself daily.

Essentially, you still eat the Ketogenic Mediterranean Diet but are adding a daily carb serving. If you have unwanted weight gain, or your weight loss progress stalls, you've added too many carbs and must cut back, or try different carb sources.

On the other hand, if you handled the extra carb serving without trouble for a week, you may add one more daily carb serving. Monitor your progress for another week.

If you're handling those carbs, you may increase by one additional carb serving every week. You've added too much carb if you gain unwanted weight, or your weight loss progress stalls. Then you must cut back or try different carbs—especially different carb groups.

Many people who have weight management problems will not be able to increase carbs to more than six additional daily servings. But that's OK because you don't necessarily need more carbs for a long and healthy life. For many folks, additional carbs are unhealthy.

By the way, if you wish to cut back on your animal protein consumption at this point, feel free. It's your choice. I'd continue to eat cold-water fatty fish at least two or three times weekly, along with the usual olive oil and nuts.

Are you with me so far?

WHICH CARBS TO ADD

OK, so you're going to add some carbs to your diet, but which ones? For the potential health benefits, I'd add carbs in this order:
- fruits
- vegetables
- whole grains
- legumes
- yogurt and other dairy products

This is just a loose guideline, not a commandment. I suggest everyone eventually add one or two servings of fruit daily, classic fruits rather than technical fruits like tomato and avocado already on the KMD. Legumes, yogurt, and other dairy products are listed after fruits and veggies because the evidence in favor of their long-term health benefits is not as strong. Eating a couple servings of whole grain daily is fairly consistently linked to a reduced risk of heart disease.

Yogurt deserves special mention because it's a component of the traditional doctor-recommended Mediterranean diet. It's a great source of calcium, a critical mineral for healthy bones, nerves, and muscles. Does it have anything special you couldn't get elsewhere? Probably not.

Now you're ready to enhance the KMD with an extra carb serving daily. Why not start with a fruit? Choose a variety of items within any given carb group, and try eventually to eat from multiple carb groups. Variety ensures you get adequate vitamins, minerals, and phytonutrients.

Nevertheless, just to be sure, continue your supplements as on the KMD. If you're sick of taking them, drop the calcium first, potassium second, then magnesium. Wait a couple weeks between each discontinuation, and monitor how you feel. Any weakness? Fatigue? Muscle cramps? Restart the dropped supplement and see if it resolves the issue.

Once your total daily digestible carb grams are up in the 60–100 g range, you have my blessing to start dropping some of the supplements you've been taking, one supplement every week or two as above.

Vitamin D is special. If you don't get much sun exposure, I'd continue to take 1,000 IU daily, indefinitely. See what your own doctor thinks. You might also benefit from ongoing daily supplementation with a multivitamin.

Things are getting a little complicated now. If you regain lost fat weight, you can always return to home base: the Ketogenic Mediterranean Diet.

Table 11.1 Carb Groups and Serving Sizes for the Low-Carb Mediterranean Diet

---

(Each serving has about 7.5 grams of digestible carbohydrate.)

Fruits

apple, a third of medium-sized one (54 g)
banana, one third (39 g)
peach, ½ of medium (75 g)
strawberry halves, two thirds of a cup (75 g)
blueberries, ½ cup (75 g)
raspberries, 1 cup (123 g)
blackberries, 1 cup (144 g)
cantaloupe, ½ cup cubes (80 g)
honeydew, 1 cup of cubes (85 g)
date, medjool, ½ date (12 g)
orange, navel, ½ (70 g)
pear, a third of medium-sized one (60 g)
pomegranate, ¼ of 4" (10 cm) diameter fruit (70g)
tangerine, ½ (44 g)
grapefruit, ½ (61 g)
cherries, sweet, raw, a third of a cup (45 g)
grapes, a third of a cup (50 g)
raisins, seedless, 20 (9 g)
nectarine, medium, ½ (70 g)
mango, slices, a third of a cup (55 g)
pineapple, raw chunks, a third of a cup (55g)
lime/lemon juice, raw, 2 limes or lemons (88 g)
watermelon, diced, two thirds of a cup (100 g)

Vegetables and Fruits

potato, white, raw, flesh and skin,
    ¼ of medium potato (53 g)
corn, canned, drained, ¼ cup (41g)
carrots, raw, strips or slices, ¾ cup (92 g)
sweet potato, raw, a third of 5 inch-long (13 cm)
    tater (45 g)
beets, canned, drained solids, ¾ cup slices (130 g)
peas, green, canned or frozen, ½ cup (67 g)
spaghetti squash, cooked, 1 cup (155 g)
KMD mixed veggies, 7 oz (200 g)

Legumes

peas, split, mature seeds, cooked/boiled,
    ¼ cup (49 g)
peas, black-eyed (cowpeas), canned, ¼ cup (60 g)
soybeans, mature seeds, roasted, 1.5 oz (42 g)
soybeans, mature seeds, cooked/boiled,
    1 cup (170 g)
beans, mature seeds, cooked/boiled, ¼ cup (43 g)
    (beans = black, kidney, navy, pinto, white, fava,
    chickpeas/garbanzo)

Yogurt and Milk Products

yogurt, plain whole milk, ½ cup
milk, whole, ½ cup
milk, 1% milk fat, ½ cup
Fage Greek, "total 2%", ½ cup (get full-fat version
    if available)
Voskos plain original Greek yogurt, ½ cup

Grains

bread, whole wheat, ½ slice (15 g)
bread, Ezekiel 4:19, ½ slice
pasta, 100% whole grain, dry, 12 g
Ry-Krisp crackers, 4.5 x 2.5" (11 x 6 cm) (11 g)
Triscuit crackers x 3 (14 g)
cracker, whole wheat, 14 g
tortilla (Mission), 8" (20 cm) whole grain,
    a third of a tortilla (16 g)
oats, dry whole grain, a third of a cup uncooked
    (13 g)
oats, steel-cut, uncooked, 1.3 tbsp (13 g)
rice, brown, cooked, 3 tbsp
quinoa, cooked, 3 tbsp (35 g)
barley, pearled, cooked, 3 tbsp (30g)
shredded wheat, plain, sugar-free (11 g)
cereal, FiberOne, original, plain,
    a third of a cup or 5 tbsp (75 ml)
Kellogg's All-Bran original or
    All-Bran Bran Buds, ¼ cup (15 g)

Table 11.1 Carb Groups and Serving Sizes
for the Low-Carb Mediterranean Diet

FOR YOUR CONVENIENCE . . .

You can print a copy of the Carb Groups and Serving Sizes from this web page:
http://advancedmediterraneandiet.com/printabledocuments.html
You'll also find a grocery shopping list for the both the KMD and LCMD at the same page.

Welcome to the Low-Carb Mediterranean Diet!

ADVANCED MEDITERRANEAN DIET: TRANSITION TO MAINTENANCE PHASE

This section is for you if you've been following the Advanced Mediterranean Diet and have reached your goal weight.

In a nutshell, my maintenance phase prescription for you is: Keep exercising, and eat a little more.

Keep exercising, and eat a little more. If you've not been exercising, start. Go out of your way to be physically active for 30 to 45 minutes on at least four days a week, if not all. Walking is fine. More vigorous activity and strength training are even better. The more you exercise, the more you can eat without getting fat again.

My advice to "eat a little more" got your attention, I suspect. But what to eat? In order to more closely approximate the health-promoting Mediterranean diet, eat more fruits, vegetables, nuts, whole grains, and olive oil. Eat more, but no too much—only a couple or three hundred calories daily, at most. That's not as much food as you think.

Eat more fruits, vegetables, nuts, whole grains, and olive oil. But not much more or you'll get fat again. You don't need any additional meat or milk products.

Among the healthy oils, olive oil has the most scientific evidence to support its consumption. Canola, soybean, and flaxseed oils are considered relatively healthy, while not part of the traditional Mediterranean diet. You should be fine substituting them for olive oil now and then.

THREE OPTIONS FOR TRANSITION

At the end of your weight-loss phase and the beginning of the maintenance phase, it is surprisingly easy to start overeating. Forewarned is forearmed. Avoid this landmine by choosing one of three options for transitioning into the maintenance phase.

The best option is to continue monitoring food and exercise on your daily log, while eating an additional 200 or 300 calories per day of various fruits, veggies, nuts, whole grains, and olive oil. Continue choosing foods from the Food Choices & Serving Sizes list, and mark them on your daily log. The calorie counts are on both documents. Continue weighing daily. Keep exercising. After a month or two of this regimen, you'll have an intuitive sense of what and how much you should be eating without regaining weight. Then stop the daily log routine.

Another transition option would be to move from your current calorie level diet to the one next higher. For example, if you lost your weight on the 1,500 calorie diet, go to the 1,900 calorie plan and fill in those daily logs for one or two months. The log will count and limit your calories for you. But as mentioned already, you truly don't need additional meat and milk products. Continue your exercise program and daily weights during this one or two month transition.

The third option for transition to the maintenance phase: if you've been exercising regularly but loathe it, you could stop exercising and stay on your current calorie level diet. See what happens with your weight. You could probably eat an extra 100 to 200 daily calories without gaining weight. Choose extra fruits, veggies, nuts, whole grains, or olive oil. Continue recording your daily intake and weight for a couple months.

In any case, do not return to eating commercially prepared concentrated sugars and refined starches on a regular basis as in the old days. No soda pop, sugar-laden sports drinks, muffins, cookies, potato chips, corn chips, pizza, etc.

At this point you can stop your multivitamin/multimineral supplement. Your body makes vitamin D if you give it adequate sun exposure. Unless you're sure you get enough sun, you may benefit from a vitamin D supplement, 1,000 IU daily for the rest of your life. Taking a calcium supplement without also taking extra D is probably not a good idea.

Weigh yourself daily during the first two months of your maintenance phase. After that, weigh at least weekly. Daily weights will remind you how hard you worked to achieve your goal. When you look now at a brownie, candy bar, or piece of pie, you ask yourself, "Do I really want to walk an extra hour or jog an extra three miles today to burn off those calories?" If so, enjoy. Otherwise, forego the unneeded calories.

WHAT IF I GAIN A LITTLE BACK?

Be aware that you might regain five or 10 pounds (two to four kg) of fat now and then. You probably will. It's not the end of the world. It's human nature. You're not a failure; you're human. But draw the line and get back on your old weight-loss program for one or two months.

Analyze and learn from the episode. Why did it happen? Slipping back into your old ways? Slacking off on exercise? Too many special occasion feasts? Allowing junk food back into the house?

Learn which food item is your nemesis—the food that consistently torpedoes your resolve to eat right. For example, I have two: candy and sweet baked goods such as cookies and muffins. If I just look at them I add a pound. Remember an old ad campaign for a potato chip: "Betcha can't eat just one!"? Well, I can't eat just one cookie. So I don't get started. I might eat one if it's the last one available. Or I satisfy my sweet craving with fresh fruit or a diet soda. Just as a recovering alcoholic can't drink any alcohol, perhaps you should totally abstain from...? You know your own personal gastronomic Achilles heel. Experiment with various strategies for vanquishing your nemesis.

It's OK to overindulge in food infrequently (10–12 times per year), on special occasions such as birthdays, wedding anniversaries, holidays. But you must counteract the extra calories by cutting down intake or by exercising more, either before or after the feast.

TWO SECRETS TO KEEPING THE WEIGHT OFF

The true measure of a successful weight management program is not simply how much weight is lost, but whether the lost weight stays lost over the long run. What distinguishes weight losers who keep the weight off from those who gain it back? Two factors, mostly:

1. Restrained eating
2. Regular physical activity

"Successful losers" apply self-restraint on an almost daily basis, avoiding food they know will lead to weight regain. They limit how much they eat. They consciously choose not to return to their old eating habits, despite urges to the contrary.

The other glaring difference is that, compared to regainers, the successful losers are physically active. Oftentimes, they exercised while losing weight, and almost always continue to exercise in the maintenance phase of their program. This is true in at least eight out of 10 cases. It's clear that regular exercise isn't always needed, but it dramatically increases your chances of long-term success.

THE PAYOFF

Congratulations, in advance perhaps, on accomplishing a worthwhile, difficult goal through Mediterranean-style eating! You now know how your body uses various nutrients and energy, and how to apply that knowledge to optimize your health and longevity. You now know that excess body fat and certain nutrients contribute to disease. Other specific nutrients promote health. You now know how to build a social support system to assist in your weight control endeavor. This knowledge base motivated you to persevere when you were tempted to abandon the effort. Your careful attention to the daily logs has confirmed and reinforced your discipline. The transformation to your slimmer body required commitment and willpower, which you may have thought at one time were in short supply. You no longer live to eat, but eat to live.

Now, be wise and do something great for those around you with your renewed vigor and longer life.

KEY POINTS

- Get real about weight gain. You can never again eat all you want, whenever you want, over sustained periods of time.
- Recognize which food item is your nemesis. Devise a strategy to overcome it.
- "Successful losers" who don't regain the weight share two characteristics: 1) restrained eating habits, and 2) regular physical activity.
- Most diets ultimately fail in the long run simply because people go back to their old habits. If you return to what you always did, you'll keep getting what you always got: gradual weight gain.
- As you enter your "maintenance of weight loss phase" after the Advanced Mediterranean Diet, the best option is to keep exercising and simply add 200–300 calories per day of fruits, vegetables, nuts, whole grains, or olive oil. Additional meat and milk products are not needed.
- In transitioning from the Ketogenic Mediterranean Diet to the Low-Carb Mediterranean Diet, carbohydrates must be added slowly and incrementally.
- Many people will not be successful at weight management if they eat over 80–100 grams of digestible carbohydrates daily.
- Continue careful monitoring of your food intake and exercise during the first two months of your maintenance phase.
- Weigh yourself daily during the first two months of your maintenance phase. After that, weigh at least weekly for the rest of your life.

- You might regain five or 10 pounds (two or four kg) now and then. If so, simply return to your previously successful weight-loss diet for one to two months. No big deal.

RECOMMENDED FURTHER READING

Books

Bittman, Mark. *How to Cook Everything: 2,000 Simple Recipes for Great Food.* Wiley, 2008.

Cloutier, Marissa and Adamson, Eve. *The Mediterranean Diet* (revised and updated). Avon Books, 2004.

Cook's Illustrated. *The New Best Recipes.* America's Test Kitchen, 2004.

Crocker, Betty. Betty *Crocker Cookbook: 1500 Recipes for the Way You Cook Today.* Betty Crocker, 2011.

Eloff, Jennifer; Emmerich, Maria; Ketchum, Carolyn; Marshall, Lisa; and Altena, Kent. *Low-Carbing Among Friends,* volume 1. Eureka Publishing, 2011.

Jenkins, Nancy Harmon. *The New Mediterranean Diet Cookbook: A Delicious Alternative for Lifelong Health.* Bantam, 2008.

Rombauer, Irma S.; Becker, Marion Rombauer; and Becker, Ethan. *Joy of Cooking: 75th Anniversary Edition.* Scribner, 2006

Taubes, Gary. *Why We Get Fat: And What to Do About It.* Knopf, 2011.

Volek, Jeff and Phinney, Stephen. *The Art and Science of Low Carbohydrate Living: An Expert Guide to Making the Life-Saving Benefits of Carbohydrate Restriction Sustainable and Enjoyable.* Beyond Obesity LLC, 2011.

Westman, Eric; Phinney, Stephen; and Volek, Jeff. *The New Atkins for a New You: The Ultimate Diet for Shedding Weight and Feeling Great.* Fireside, 2010.

Whitney, Eleanor Noss and Rolfes, Sharon Rady. *Understanding Nutrition* (10th edition). Wadsworth Publishing Company, 2010.

Wright, Clifford A. *A Mediterranean Feast.* William Morrow Ccokbooks, 1999.

Recommended Further Reading

Internet

About.com: Low Carb Diets. Guide: Laura Dolson
http://lowcarbdiets.about.com/

All Day I Dream About Food (low-carb recipes by Carolyn)
http://dreamaboutfood.blogspot.com/

Allrecipes.com
http://www.allrecipes.com
"Devoted to a community of home cooks," this site has over 30,000 free recipes with detailed nutritional analysis, including calories per serving. Numerous Mediterranean-style dishes (enter search word "Mediterranean").

Clifford A. Wright
http://www.cliffordawright.com
This cook and writer specializes in regional cuisines of the Mediterranean region, with emphasis on culinary history. You will find some recipes here along with historical articles and numerous helpful Internet links.

DARdreams (low-carb recipes)
http://dardreams.wordpress.com/

Fat Head by Tom Naughton (low-carb lifestyle)
http://www.fathead-movie.com/

Hold the Toast! by Dana Carpender (low-carb lifestyle)
http://holdthetoast.com/

Jimmy Moore's Livin' La Vida Low Carb Blog (renowned low-carb advocate)
http://livinlavidalowcarb.com/blog/

Oldways Preservation and Exchange Trust
http://www.oldwayspt.org
This nonprofit "food issues think tank" facilitates the translation of nutrition science into practical healthy eating patterns, including the traditional Mediterranean diet.

Physical Activity for Everyone
http://www.cdc.gov/nccdphp/dnpa/physical/

Recipezaar
http://www.recipezaar.com
Need a recipe for whole wheat pancakes? You'll find several at this free site, among the 200,000 other recipes and 13,000 cookbooks. The recipes are rated by website users who have prepared

the dishes submitted for publication by other users. Most recipes are provided with nutritional analysis

Shape Up America!
http://www.shapeup.org
"Founded in 1994, Shape Up America! is a 501(c)3 not-for-profit organization committed to raising awareness of obesity as a health issue and to providing responsible information on healthy weight management."

Splendid Low-Carbing by Jennifer Eloff (low-carb recipes)
http://low-carb-news.blogspot.com/

The Blog of Michael R. Eades, M.D. (renowned low-carb advocate and co-author of *Protein Power*)
http://proteinpower.com/drmike/

The Whole Grains Council
http://www.wholegrainscouncil.org
Learn more about the benefits of various whole grains and how to find whole grain products. Many recipes here, plus links to hundreds of recipes at other sites.

Weight-Control Information Network
http://www.win.niddk.nih.gov/index.htm
A service of the (U.S.) National Institute of Diabetes and Digestive and Kidney Diseases. Information for the public and healthcare professionals on obesity, weight control, related nutritional matters, and physical activity.

SELECTED REFERENCES BY TOPIC

Topics

Dietary Fat Doesn't Cause Heart and Vascular
  Disease
Rationale for the Advanced Mediterranean
  Diet
Superior Effectiveness of Low-Carb Dieting

You can read most of the following articles or their abstracts on-line at the publishing journal's website.

Dietary Fat Doesn't Cause Heart and Vascular Disease

Siri-Tarino, Patty, et al. Meta-analysis of prospective cohort studies evaluating the association of saturated fat with cardiovascular disease. *American Journal of Clinical Nutrition*, January 13, 2010. doi:10.3945/ajcn.2009.27725

Skeaff, C. Murray and Miller, Jody. Dietary fat and coronary heart disease: Summary of evidence from prospective cohort and randomised controlled trials. *Annals of Nutrition and Metabolism*, 55 (2009): 173–201.

Halton, Thomas, et al. Low-carbohydrate-diet score and the risk of coronary heart disease in women. *New England Journal of Medicine,* 355 (2006): 1,991–2,002.

German, J. Bruce, and Dillard, Cora J. Saturated fats: What dietary intake? *American Journal of Clinical Nutrition*, 80 (2004): 550–559.

Ravnskov, U. The questionable role of saturated and polyunsaturated fatty acids in cardiovascular disease. *Journal of Clinical Epidemiology*, 51 (1998): 443–460.

Ravsnskov, U. Hypothesis out-of-date. The diet-heart idea. *Jour-*

nal of Clinical Epidemiology, 55 (2002): 1,057–1,063.

Ravnskov, U, et al. Studies of dietary fat and heart disease. Science, 295 (2002): 1,464-1,465.

Taubes, G. The soft science of dietary fat. Science, 291 (2001): 2,535–2,541.

Zarraga, Ignatius, and Schwartz, Ernst. Impact of dietary patterns and interventions on cardiovascular health. Circulation, 114 (2006): 961–973.

Mente, Andrew, et al. A Systematic Review of the Evidence Supporting a Causal Link Between Dietary Factors and Coronary Heart Disease. Archives of Internal Medicine, 169 (2009): 659–669.

Parikh, Parin, et al. Diets and cardiovascular disease: an evidence-based assessment. Journal of the American College of Cardiology, 45 (2005): 1,379–1,387.

Hooper, L., et al. Dietary fat intake and prevention of cardiovascular disease: systematic review. British Medical Journal, 322 (2001): 757-763.

Weinberg, W.C. The Diet-Heart Hypothesis: a critique. Journal of the American College of Cardiology, 43 (2004): 731–733.

Mozaffarian, Darius, et al. Dietary fats, carbohydrate, and progression of coronary atherosclerosis in postmenopausal women. American Journal of Clinical Nutrition, 80 (2004): 1,175–1,184.

Knopp, Robert and Retzlaff, Barbara. Saturated fat prevents coronary artery disease? An American paradox. American Journal of Clinical Nutrition, 80 (2004): 1,102–1,103.

Yusuf, S., et al. Effect of potentially modifiable risk factors associated with myocardial infarction in 52 countries (the INTERHEART study): case-control study. Lancet, 364 (2004): 937–952. (ApoB/ApoA1 ratio was a risk factor for heart attack, so dietary saturated fat may play a role if it affects this ratio.)

Hu, Frank. Diet and cardiovascular disease prevention: The need for a paradigm shift. Journal of the American College of Cardiology, 50 (2007): 22–24.

Oh, K., et al. Dietary fat intake and risk of coronary heart disease in women: 20 years of follow-up of the Nurses' Health Study. American Journal of Epidemiology, 161 (2005): 672–679.

Rationale for the Advanced Mediterranean Diet

Ronksley, P.E., et al. Association of alcohol consumption with selected cardiovascular disease outcomes: a systematic review and meta-analysis. British Medical Journal, 342 (2011). PMID: 21343207.

Scarmeas, N., et al. Mediterranean diet and magnetic resonance imaging-assessed cerebrovascular disease. Annals of Neurol-

ogy, 69 (2011): 257-268. doi: 10.1002/ana.22317

Sofi, F., et al. Accruing evidence about benefits of adherence to the Mediterranean diet on health: an updated systematic review and meta-analysis. *The American Journal of Clinical Nutrition* (2010). PMID: 20810976.

Chrysohoou, C., et al. The Mediterranean diet contributes to the preservation of left ventricular systolic function and to the long-term favorable prognosis of patients who have had an acute coronary event. *American Journal of Clinical Nutrition* (2010). doi: 10.3945/ajcn.2009.28982.

Ding, E.L, and Mozaffarian, D. Optimal dietary habits for the prevention of stroke. *Seminars in Neurology*, 26 (2006): 11-23.

Sabaté, Joan and Ang, Yen. Nuts and health outcomes: New epidemiologic evidence. *American Journal of Clinical Nutrition*, 89 (2009): 1,643S-1,648S.

Fung, Teresa, et al. Mediterranean diet and incidence of and mortality from coronary heart disease and stroke in women. *Circulation*, 119 (2009): 1,093-1,100.

Mente, Andrew, et al. A systematic review of the evidence supporting a causal link between dietary factors and coronary heart disease. *Archives of Internal Medicine, 169 (2009): 659-669.*

Salas-Salvado, Jordi, et al. Effect of a Mediterranean diet supplemented with nuts on metabolic syndrome status: One-year results of the PREDIMED randomized trial. *Archives of Internal Medicine*, 168 (2008): 2,449-2,458.

King, Dana E., et al. Adopting moderate alchohol consumption in middle age: Subsequent cardiovascular events. *American Journal of Medicine*, 121 (2008): 201-206.

Mellen, Philip, et al. Whole grain intake and cardiovascular disease: A meta-analysis. *Nutrition, Metabolism & Cardiovascular Diseases*, 18, (2008): 283-290.

Mitrou, Panagiota N., et al. Mediterranean dietary pattern and prediction of all-cause mortality in a US population. *Archives of Internal Medicine*, 167 (2007): 2461-2468.

Tangney, C.C., et al. Adherence to a Mediterranean-type dietary pattern and cognitive decline in a community population. *American Journal of Clinical Nutrition*, 93 (2011): 601-607.

Bendinelli, B., et al. Fruit, vegetables, and olive oil and risk of coronary heart disease in Italian women: the EPICOR Study. *American Journal of Clinical Nutrition*, 93 (2011): 275-283.

Kastorinin, C.M., et al. The effect of Mediterranean diet on metabolic syndrome and its components: a meta- analysis of 50 studies and 534,906 individuals. *Journal of the American College of Cardiology*, 57 (2011): 1,299-1,313.

Mares, J.A., et al. Healthy lifestyles related to subsequent prevalence of age-related macular degeneration. *Archives of Ophthalmology*, 129 (2011): 470-480.

Albanese, Emiliano, et al. Dietary fish and meat intake and dementia in Latin America, China, and India: a 10/66 Dementia Research Group population-based study. *American Journal of Clinical Nutrition*, 90 (2009): 392-400.

Feart, Catherine, et al. Adherence to a Mediterranean diet, cognitive decline, and risk of dementia. *Journal of the American Medical Association*, 302 (2009): 638-648.

Scarmeas, Nikolaos, et al. Physical activity, diet, and risk of Alzheimer Disease. *Journal of the American Medical Association*, 302 (2009): 627-637.

Scarmeas, Nikolaos, et al. Mediterranean diet and mild cognitive impairment. *Archives of Neurology*, 66 (2009): 216-225.

Trichopoulou, A., et al. Conformity to traditional Mediterranean diet and breast cancer risk in the Greek EPIC (European Prospective Investigation into Cancer and nutrition) cohort. *American Journal of Clinical Nutrition* (2010). doi: 10.3945/ajcn.2010.29619.

Buckland, Genevieve, et al. Adherence to a Mediterranean diet and risk of gastric adenocarcinoma within the European Prospective Investigation into Cancer and Nutrition (EPIC) cohort study. *American Journal of Clinical Nutrition*, (2009). doi: 10.3945/ajcn.2009.28209.

Benetou, V., et al. Conformity to traditional Mediterranean diet and cancer incidence: the Greek EPIC cohort. *British Journal of Cancer*, 99 (2008): 191-195.

Salas-Salvado, J., et al. Reduction in the incidence of type 2-diabetes with the Mediterranean diet: Results of the PREDIMED-Reus Nutrition Intervention Randomized Trial. *Diabetes Care*, (2010). doi: 10.2337/dc10-1288.

Baliunas, D.O., et al. Alcohol as a risk factor for type 2 diabetes: A systematic review and meta-analysis. *Diabetes Care*, 32 (2009): 2,123-2,132.

Barclay, Alan W., et al. Glycemic index, glycemic load, and chronic disease risk - a meta-analysis of observational studies [of mostly women]. *American Journal of Clinical Nutrition*, 87 (2008): 627-637.

Shai, Iris, et al. Weight Loss with a Low-Carbohydrate, Mediterranean, or Low-Fat Diet. *New England Journal of Medicine*, 359 (2008): 229-241.

Mozaffarian, Dariush, et al. Incidence of new-onset diabetes and impaired fasting glucose in patients with recent myocardial infarction and the effect of clinical and lifestyle risk factors. *Lancet*, 370 (2007): 667-675.

Martinez-Gonzalez, M.A., et al. Adherence to Mediterranean diet and risk of developing diabetes: prospective cohort study. *British Medical Journal*, 336 (7657)(2008): 1,348-1,351.

Barros, R., et al. Adherence to the Mediterranean diet and fresh fruit intake are associated with improved asthma control. *Allergy*, 63 (2008): 917-923.

King, Dana E., et al. Adopting Moderate Alchohol Consumption in Middle Age: Subsequent Cardiovascular Events. *American Journal of Medicine*, 121 (2008): 201-206.

Albert, Christine, et al. Nut consumption and decreased risk of sudden cardiac death in the Physicians' Health Study. *Archives of Internal Medicine*, 162 (2002): 1,382-1,387.

Alpert, Joseph S. What diet should we recommend to patients? [editorial]. *American Journal of Medicine*, 119 (2006): 715-716.

Brunner, Eric. Oily fish and omega 3 fat supplements [editorial]. *British Medical Journal*, 332 (2006): 739-740.

GISSI-Prevenzione Investigators. Dietary supplementation with n-3 polyunsaturated fatty acids [eicosapentaenoic acid and docosahexaenoic acid] and vitamin E after myocardial infarction: results of the GISSI-Prevenzione trial. *Lancet*, 354 (1999): 447-455.

Hooper, Lee, et al. Risks and benefits of omega 3 fats for mortality, cardiovascular disease, and cancer: systematic review. *British Medical Journal*, 332 (2006): 752-760.

Keys, Ancel. *Seven Countries: A Multivariate Analysis of Death and Coronary Artery Disease.* Harvard University Press, 1980.

Keys, Ancel and Keys, Margaret. *How to Eat Well and Stay Well the Mediterranean Way.* Doubleday, 1975.

Keys, Ancel. Coronary heart disease in seven countries. *Circulation*, 41, (1970) supplement I: I-1 through I-211.

Knoops, Kim T.B., et al. Mediterranean diet, lifestyle factors, and 10-year mortality in elderly European men and women: The HALE Project. *Journal of the American Medical Association*, 292 (2004): 1,433-1,439.

Kushi, Lawrence H., et al. American Cancer Society guidelines on nutrition and physical activity for cancer prevention: Reducing the risk of cancer with healthy food choices and physical activity. *CA: A Cancer Journal for Clinicians*, 56 (2006): 254-281.

Lorgeril, M., et al. Mediterranean diet, traditional risk factors, and the rate of cardiovascular complications after myocardial infarction: Final report of the Lyon Diet Heart Study. *Circulation*, 99 (1999): 779-785.

Mozaffarian, Dariush and Rimm, Eric B. Fish intake, contaminants, and human health: Evaluating the risks and the benefits. *Journal of the American Medical Association*, 296 (2006): 1,885-1,899.

Superior Effectiveness of Low-Carb Dieting

Brehm, B.J., et al. A randomized trial comparing a very low carbohydrate diet and a calorie-restricted low fat diet on body weight and cardiovascular risk factors in healthy women. Journal *of Clinical Endocrinology and Metabolism*, 88 (2003): 1,617–1,623.

Samaha, F.F., et al. A low-carbohydrate as compared with a low-fat diet in severe obesity. *New England Journal of Medicine*, 348 (2003): 2,074–2,081.

Sondike, S.B., et al. Effects of a low-carbohydrate diet on weight loss and cardiovascular risk factor in overweight adolescents. *Journal of Pediatrics*, 143 (2003): 253–258.

Aude, Y.W., et al. The National Cholesterol Education Program diet versus a diet lower in carbohydrates and higher in protein and monounsaturated fat. A randomized trial. *Archives of Internal Medicine*, 164 (2004): 2,141–2,146.

Volek, J.S., et al. Comparison of energy-restricted very low-carbohydrate and low-fat diets on weight loss and body composition in overweight men and women. *Nutrition & Metabolism*, 1 (2004), 1:13.

Yancy, W.S. Jr, et al. A low-carbohydrate, ketogenic diet versus a low-fat diet to treat obesity and hyperlipidemia. A randomized, controlled trial. *Annals of Internal Medicine*, 140 (2004): 769–777.

Nichols-Richardsson, S.M., et al. Perceived hunger is lower and weight loss is greater in overweight premenopausal women consuming a low-carbohydrate/high- protein versus high-carbohydrate/low-fat diet. *Journal of the American Dietetic Association*, 105 (205): 1,433–1,437.

Gardner, C.D., et al. Comparison of the Atkins, Zone, Ornish, and learn diets for change in weight and related risk factors among overweight premenopausal women. The A to Z Weight Loss Study: A randomized trial. *Journal of the American Medical Association*, 297 (2007): 969–977.

Shai, I., et al. Weight loss with a low-carbohydrate, Mediterranean, or low-fat diet. *New England Journal of Medicine*, 359 (2008): 229–241.

Dyson, P.A., et al. A low-carbohydrate diet is more effective in reducing body weight than healthy eating in both diabetic and non-diabetic subjects. *Diabetic Medicine*, 24 (2007): 1,430–1,435.

Krebs, N.F., et al. Efficacy and safety of a high protein, low carbohydrate diet for weight loss in severely obese adolescents. Journal of Pediatrics, 157 (2010): 252–258.

Summer, S.S., et al. Adiponectin changes in relation to the macronutrient composition of a weight-loss diet. *Obesity*, (March 31, 2011). doi: 10.1038/oby.2011.60.

Daly, M.E., et al. Short-term effects of severe dietary carbohydrate-restriction advice in type 2 diabetes. A randomized controlled trial. *Diabetes Medicine*, 23 (2006): 15–20.

Westman, E.C., et al. The effect of a low carbohydrate,

293

ketogenic diet versus a low-glycemic index diet on glycemic control in type 2 diabetes mellitus. *Nutrition and Metabolism,* 5 (2008): 36 (December 19).

RECIPE INDEX

Ketogenic Mediterranean Diet

Advanced Mediterranean diet

Recipe Index